Translational Medicine
Strategies and Statistical Methods

Chapman & Hall/CRC Biostatistics Series

Editor-in-Chief

Shein-Chung Chow, Ph.D.
Professor
Department of Biostatistics and Bioinformatics
Duke University School of Medicine
Durham, North Carolina, U.S.A.

Series Editors

Byron Jones
Senior Director
Statistical Research and Consulting Centre
(IPC 193)
Pfizer Global Research and Development
Sandwich, Kent, UK

Jen-pei Liu
Professor
Division of Biometry
Department of Agronomy
National Taiwan University
Taipei, Taiwan

Karl E. Peace
Georgia Cancer Coalition
Distinguished Cancer Scholar
Senior Research Scientist and
Professor of Biostatistics
Jiann-Ping Hsu College of Public Health
Georgia Southern University
Statesboro, GA

Bruce W. Turnbull
Professor
School of Operations Research
and Industrial Engineering
Cornell University
Ithaca, NY

Chapman & Hall/CRC Biostatistics Series

Published Titles

Chapman & Hall/CRC Biostatistics Series

Translational Medicine
Strategies and Statistical Methods

Edited by

Dennis Cosmatos
Wyeth Research
Collegeville, Pennsylvania, U.S.A.

Shein-Chung Chow
Duke University School of Medicine
Durham, North Carolina, U.S.A.

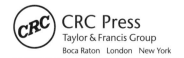

CRC Press
Taylor & Francis Group
Boca Raton London New York

CRC Press is an imprint of the
Taylor & Francis Group, an **informa** business

A CHAPMAN & HALL BOOK

Chapman & Hall/CRC
Taylor & Francis Group
6000 Broken Sound Parkway NW, Suite 300
Boca Raton, FL 33487-2742

© 2009 by Taylor & Francis Group, LLC
Chapman & Hall/CRC is an imprint of Taylor & Francis Group, an Informa business

No claim to original U.S. Government works
Printed in the United States of America on acid-free paper
10 9 8 7 6 5 4 3 2 1

International Standard Book Number-13: 978-1-58488-872-7 (Hardcover)

Library of Congress Cataloging-in-Publication Data

Translational medicine : strategies and statistical methods / edited by Dennis
    Cosmatos and Shein-Chung Chow.
        p. cm.
    Includes bibliographical references and index.
    ISBN-13: 978-1-58488-872-7
    ISBN-10: 1-58488-872-5
    1. Medical innovations. 2. Medicine--Research--Statistical methods. 3.
Biochemical markers. 4. Drug development. I. Cosmatos, Dennis. II. Chow,
Shein-Chung, 1955- III. Title.

RA418.5.M4T73 2009
610.72'7--dc22   2008045100

Visit the Taylor & Francis Web site at
http://www.taylorandfrancis.com

and the CRC Press Web site at
http://www.crcpress.com

Contents

Preface

In recent years, the concept of translational medicine (or translational research) to expedite clinical research and development has attracted much attention. Translational medicine (TM) is referred to as the translation of basic research discoveries into clinical applications. More specifically, translational research takes the discoveries from basic research to a patient and measures an endpoint in a patient. Basically, translational research or TM encompasses not only the identification and validation of clinically relevant biomarkers, but also the conduct of nonhuman and nonclinical studies with the intent of developing principles for the discovery of new therapeutic strategies. The goals of translational research or TM are essentially no different from those of traditional clinical research. TM emphasizes strategies to expedite their successful implementation.

From an operational view, TM is a multidisciplinary entity that bridges basic scientific research with clinical development. As developing therapeutic pharmaceutical compounds become more expensive and the success rates for getting such compounds approved for marketing and getting them to the patients in need of these treatments continue to decrease, a focused effort has emerged in improving the communication and planning between basic and clinical science. This will likely lead to more therapeutic insights being derived from new scientific ideas, and more feedback being provided to research so that their approaches are better targeted. TM spans all the disciplines and activities that lead to making key scientific decisions as a compound traverses across the difficult preclinical–clinical divide. Many argue that improvement in making correct decisions on what dose and regimen should be pursued in the clinic; the likely human safety risks of a compound, the likely drug interactions, and the pharmacologic behavior of the compound are the most important decisions made in the entire development process. Many of these decisions and the path for uncovering this information within later development are defined at this specific time within the drug development process. Improving these decisions will likely lead to a substantial increase in the number of safe and effective compounds available to combat human diseases.

As indicated by Mankoff et al. (2004), there are three major obstacles to effective TM in practice. The first is the challenge of translating basic science discoveries into clinical studies. The second hurdle is the translation of clinical studies into medical practice and health care policy. The third obstacle to effective TM is philosophical. It may be unreasonable to think that basic science (without observations from the clinic and without epidemiological findings of possible associations between different diseases) will efficiently produce the novel therapies for human testing. Pilot studies such as nonhuman and nonclinical studies are often used to transition therapies developed using animal models to a clinical setting. Statisticians often assist in the planning and analysis of pilot studies. The purpose of this book is to provide a comprehensive review of statistical design and methodology that are commonly employed in translational research.

This book will aim at examining carefully each and every decision process that is critical in making a successful transition from basic science to a clinical setting. Along with a thorough review of the existing processes and disciplines that are involved in advancing a compound through the development chain, there will be a detailed discussion and development of alternative research approaches within each of those disciplines that can lead not only to faster decisions, but, most importantly, an increase in the proportion of correct decisions made on data from that research. As statistics is the primary discipline that can be applied across all research disciplines that make data-based decisions, it is natural that a research approach that incorporates a strong statistical mindset is likely to be the approach that is most likely to provide a correct conclusion from that research. We hope that the reader recognizes the value of such a mindset and carefully considers the powerful, statistically validated design and analysis approaches that are discussed.

Details of how a TM approach would impact key processes and strategies for extracting potential benefit from such changes are discussed in Chapter 2. Chapter 3 presents a detailed discussion of a variety of data types and experiments run in a productive biomarker laboratory, and discusses the optimal statistical methods for each of the specified experiments. Chapter 4 continues with the discussion on how biomarker development can impact the R&D process. Chapter 5 elaborates on how one way TM (enrichment process) can be introduced into clinical studies (target clinical trials), and Chapter 6 concentrates on some specialized statistical methods developed for studies where translational information is a key target of the study. Chapter 7 introduces nonparametric approaches to analysis of data from these translational studies, and Chapter 8 presents an approach for building, executing, and validating statistical models that consider data from various phases of development. Chapter 9 focuses on bridging studies that target clarification of relationships between numerous study endpoints, and Chapter 10 introduces a truly "translational" example where we try to find a link between 5000 year old, empirically based approaches in traditional Chinese medicine and the experiment-based approaches employed in Western medicine.

We would like to thank David Grubbs, from Taylor & Francis, for providing us the opportunity to work on this book. Dennis Cosmatos wishes to thank his wife Irene for the support and encouragement she provided him while working on this book and for being his most reliable audience for bouncing off ideas. Shein-Chung Chow wishes to express his thanks to his fiancé Annpey Pong, PhD, for her constant support and encouragement during the preparation of this book. We would like to thank our colleagues from Translational Development, Wyeth Research, and the Department of Biostatistics and Bioinformatics, Duke University School of Medicine, for their support during the preparation of this book. We wish to express our gratitude to the following individuals for their encouragement and support: Giora Feuerstein, MD and Michael E. (Ted) Burczynski, PhD, Wyeth Research; Robert Califf, MD,

Ralph Corey, MD, and John McHutchison, MD of Duke University School of Medicine; Greg Campbell, PhD of the U.S. Food and Drug Administration (U.S. FDA); Chinfu Hsiao, PhD and Walter Liu, MD of the National Health Research Institutes, Taiwan; all of the contributors, and many friends from the academia (e.g., Jen-pei Liu, PhD of National Taiwan University and Siu-Keung Tse of City University of Hong Kong), the pharmaceutical industry (e.g., Kongming Wang, PhD of Wyeth and Mark Chang, PhD of Millennium Pharmaceuticals, Inc.), and regulatory agencies (e.g., Lilly Yue, PhD, Yi Tsong, PhD, and James Hung, PhD of the U.S. FDA).

Finally, the views expressed are those of the authors and not necessarily those of Wyeth Research and Duke University School of Medicine. We are solely responsible for the contents and errors of this edition. Any comments and suggestions will be very much appreciated.

Dennis Cosmatos
Shein-Chung Chow

Contributors

Michael E. Burczynski
Biomarker Laboratory
Clinical Translational Medicine
Wyeth Research
Collegeville, Pennsylvania

Mark Chang
Biostatistics and Data Management
AMAG Pharmaceuticals, Inc.
Cambridge, Massachusetts

Herng-Der Chern
Center for Drug Evaluation
Taipei, Taiwan

Shein-Chung Chow
Department of Biostatistics
 and Bioinformatics
Duke University School
 of Medicine
Durham, North Carolina

Dennis Cosmatos
Early Development and Clinical
 Pharmacology
Wyeth Research
Collegeville, Pennsylvania

Giora Feuerstein
Discovery Translational Medicine
Wyeth Research
Collegeville, Pennsylvania

Stephen B. Forlow
Biomarker Laboratory
Clinical Translational Medicine
Wyeth Research
Collegeville, Pennsylvania

Chin-Fu Hsiao
Division of Biostatistics
 and Bioinformatics
TCOG Statistical Center
National Health Research Institutes
Zhunan, Taiwan

Jennifer A. Isler
Biomarker Laboratory
Clinical Translational Medicine
Wyeth Research
Collegeville, Pennsylvania

Zhaosheng Lin
Biomarker Laboratory
Clinical Translational Medicine
Wyeth Research
Collegeville, Pennsylvania

Jen-pei Liu
Division of Biometry
Department of Agronomy
TCOG Statistical Center
National Taiwan University
Taipei, Taiwan

 and

Division of Biostatistics
 and Bioinformatics
TCOG Statistical Center
National Health Research Institutes
Zhunan, Taiwan

Siu-Keung Tse
Department of Management Sciences
City University of Hong Kong
Hong Kong, China

Hsiao-Hui Tsou
Division of Biostatistics
 and Bioinformatics
National Health Research Institutes
Zhunan, Taiwan

Kongming Wang
Global Biostatistics and Programming
Wyeth Research
Cambridge, Massachusetts

Mey Wang
Division of Biostatistics
Center for Drug Evaluation
Taipei, Taiwan

Jessie Q. Xia
National Institute of the Statistical
 Sciences
Research Triangle Park, North Carolina

S. Stanley Young
National Institute of the Statistical
 Sciences
Research Triangle Park, North Carolina

Chapter 1

Translational Medicine: Strategies and Statistical Methods

Dennis Cosmatos and Shein-Chung Chow

Contents

1.1 Introduction: What Is Translational Medicine?

We can visualize translational medicine (TM) as an entity created from the knowledge of individuals from multiple disciplines. Being contained (formally or informally) in this single entity allows one a more harmonized approach to exchanging information and knowledge, resulting in easier and quicker availability of valuable, safe, and efficacious treatments for many diseases still affecting our population. Most directly, the practice of TM demands that early researchers look forward and completely understand how every part of their research would impact clinical development. Likewise, it requires clinical scientists to look backward and fully consider all the preclinical experiments conducted to date and continue to consider the use of going back to conduct additional experiments as and when new clinical questions arise. In particular, once relationships between preclinical and clinical results are studied and appropriate mappings are completed (e.g., dose, absorption, pharmacokinetic properties, etc.), more meaningful animal experiments can be devised. This two-directional mindset is the key to the overall approach of TM. It must be noted that for many institutions, academic and industrial, this will require substantial change in logistics and processes.

As the expense in developing therapeutic pharmaceutical compounds continues to increase and the success rate for getting such compounds approved for marketing and to the patients needing these treatments continues to decrease (see Section 1.2), a focused effort has emerged in improving the communication and planning between basic and clinical science. This will probably lead to more therapeutic insights being

1

derived from new scientific ideas, and more feedbacks being provided to researchers so that their approaches are better targeted. TM spans all the disciplines and activities that lead to making key scientific decisions, as a compound that traverses across the difficult preclinical–clinical divide. Many argue that improvement in making correct decisions on what dose and regimen should be pursued in the clinic, the anticipated human safety risks of a compound, the probable drug interactions, and the pharmacologic behavior of the compound are very likely to be the most important decisions made in the entire development process. Many of these decisions and the path for uncovering this information within later development are defined at this specific time within the drug development process. Improving these decisions will probably lead to a substantial increase in the number of safe and effective compounds available to combat human diseases.

Most inferences being made throughout the entire process are based on data. Hence, within a TM paradigm, statistics can play an extremely important role. The statistical approaches applied in TM need to draw broad conclusions from "noisy" data, typical in the discovery phase and genomic, proteomic, or other -omic data. Alternative approaches need to be used for drawing more targeted and stable conclusions from small preclinical and early clinical studies. Most importantly, statistics is best equipped to be the major "translator" in TM. In any language translation effort, it is important for the translator to know both (or several) languages that are being translated. In pharmaceutical development, the statistician is best equipped to serve this role, as he/she works across the discovery, preclinical and clinical disciplines, and implements design and analysis approaches that are well known by any properly trained statistician. Admittedly, subject knowledge and skill in applying appropriate techniques in a given discipline are needed to function effectively in each discipline, but that is attainable. A more difficult task is to develop new methods for this new discipline. This may happen once the basics are understood.

Being evident in many new technologies of the past, the statistical involvement occurs only after a field develops to a point of some analysis and design approaches (often developed without statistical input) that are being used, and then steps in to point out the error in using such techniques. Unfortunately, this has often resulted in the field progressing in lesser optimal directions, sometimes, with great reluctance to change a common practice of the past, even if it was not optimal. For example, the idea of measuring fold changes in gene expression without understanding the baseline variability for that particular gene, the use of over-parameterized linear models on -omic data that are known to be nonnormal, nonindependent, and heteroskedastic in nature, or the use of large sample testing procedures in analyzing and reporting data from preclinical experiments with sample sizes as small as $N = 3$. With all these situations, it is well known that better statistical approaches need to be adopted; however, implementing them into established disciplines is extremely difficult.

In TM, statistics, perhaps for the first time, can enter a new discipline and be part of its development at the onset of this new field, rather than being its critic and trying to repair its flaws at a later date. This text partly intends to demonstrate to the nonstatistical scientists how this can be done, and aims to guide future statisticians who will be supporting this field on how to carry out this method. In particular, the format we follow in Chapter 3 is to have a nonstatistical scientist, well entrenched in discovery translational medicine, with a clear vision of how it should proceed, providing a background and short discussion on topics of greatest value in the particular subcategory. Then, we bring together valuable statistical methods that can contribute to design and analysis knowledge to address the issues mentioned.

1.2 Why Consider TM Approaches?

To address this question, we need to take a comprehensive and objective look at the pharmaceutical industry and its common research and development (R&D) processes. As with any process, the value and success of a process is judged by its output. For the pharmaceutical industry, its output can be measured by a single solid variable: how many new drugs reach the market.

Figure 1.1 provides a glimpse of our first level of concern. The endpoint that we agreed to be a barometer of success, i.e., the number of drugs to get into the market, has been following a steady downward trend. This alone should give rise to our immediate need to examine the existing processes and try to uncover what is the cause. To compound the problem, the cost of getting each drug to the market has also gone up (Figure 1.2).

At the root of this problem is an increasing failure rate in the new compounds going through the R&D pipeline (Figure 1.3). Although the timeframes for these data differ, the observed trend continues (discussed below). It can be observed that

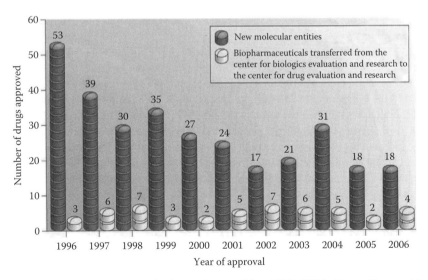

FIGURE 1.1: FDA approval of new drug entities 1996–2006. (From Owens, *Nat. Rev. Drug Discov.*, 6, 99, 2007.)

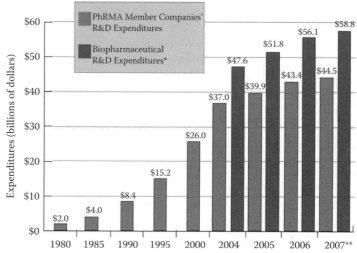

*The "Biopharmaceutical R&D" figures include PhRMA research associates
and nonmembers; these are not included in "PhRMA Member Companies'
R&D Expenditures." PhRMA first reported this data in 2004.
**Estimated.

FIGURE 1.2:   Biopharmaceutical companies' investment in R&D remains strong.
(From Pharmaceuticals and Manufacturers of America, Pharmaceutical industry profile 2008 [Washington DC: PhRMA, March 2008].)

with only a 55% success rate in phase I and 25% success rate in phase II, there is
a loss of 86% of all compounds that come into early clinical development from our
preclinical laboratories.

All these events impact not only the industry, but ultimately the society as well.
On March 2004, the United States Food and Drug Administration (FDA) released
a report, "Innovation/Stagnation: Challenge and Opportunity on the Critical Path to
New Medical Products," addressing the recent slowdown in innovative medical therapies, which is submitted to the FDA for approval. The report emphasizes the urgent
need to modernize the medical-product development process—the critical path—to
make product development more predictable and less costly. At this meeting, a senior
FDA official notified the audience that the success rate at registration had dropped
to 50% in 2003, and "most of the failures at registration (were) due to the sponsor
selecting the wrong dose or regimen for the test drug."

This serious situation led the FDA to initiate this national effort to advance medical-
product development sciences that can turn discoveries into medical miracles. FDA
took the lead in the development of a national Critical Path Opportunities List,
to bring concrete focus to these tasks. As a result, in 2006, the FDA released a
Critical Path Opportunities List that outlines 76 initial projects to bridge the gap
between the quick pace of new biomedical discoveries and the slower pace at which
those discoveries are currently developed into therapies, 2 years later (see, e.g.,

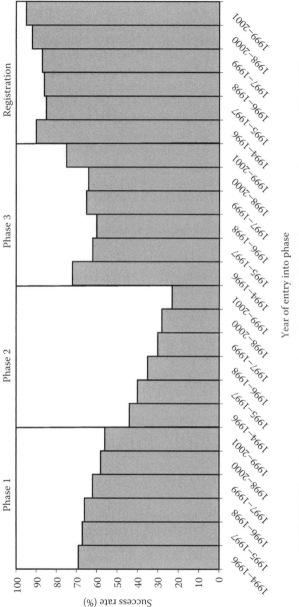

FIGURE 1.3: Success rates at various phases of clinical development between 1994–2001.

http://www.fda.gov/oc/initiatives/criticalpath). The Critical Path Opportunities List consists of six broad topic areas of (1) development of biomarkers, (2) clinical trial designs, (3) bioinformatics, (4) manufacturing, (5) public health needs, and (6) pediatrics.

As indicated in the Critical Path Opportunities Report, biomarker development is considered as the most important area for improving medical-product development. Biomarkers are measurable characteristics that reflect physiological, pharmacological, or disease processes in animals or humans. Biomarkers can reduce uncertainty by providing quantitative predictions about performance of the medical product under development. The existence of predictive biomarkers is important in expediting medical product development, because a validated biomarker, based on its response, can provide an accurate and reliable prediction of clinical performance. This process of predicting clinical performance through a validated biomarker response or based on some nonclinical or animal test results is referred to as the translational process. As a result, TM can revolutionize medical-product development in a disease area. Having observed how this mandate has been interpreted and sometimes misinterpreted (e.g., "we need to speed up the R&D process"), we aim to provide a view of TM not only as a process to utilize biomarkers, but expand it to a mindset that creates communication and knowledge-sharing across the critical nonclinical–preclinical–clinical divides.

1.3 Enhancing the Discipline of TM

In recent years, the concept of TM to expedite clinical research and development has attracted much attention. On September 8, 2005, NIH released a Notice (NOT-RM-05–013) in the NIH Guide, announcing its plan to issue two Requests for Applications (RFAs): (1) to solicit applications for Institutional Clinical and Translational Science Awards (CTSA) and (2) to solicit applications for Planning Grants for CTSAs. The purpose of the CTSA initiative, which NCRR is leading on behalf of the NIH Roadmap for Medical Research, is to assist the institutions to forge a uniquely transformative, novel, and integrative academic home for Clinical and Translational Science that has the consolidated resources to: (1) captivate, advance, and nurture a cadre of well-trained, multi- and interdisciplinary investigators and research teams; (2) create an incubator for innovative research tools and information technologies; and (3) synergize multidisciplinary and interdisciplinary clinical and translational research and researchers to catalyze the application of new knowledge and techniques to clinical practice at the frontlines of patient care.

Many pharmaceutical companies have established TM groups to facilitate the interaction between basic research and clinical medicine (particularly in clinical trials). Traditionally, basic research has been separated from the clinical practice of medicine by a series of hurdles that decreased the probability of success of promising compounds. The move toward TM is to remove these hurdles and stimulate bench-to-bedside research.

1.4 Major Obstacles of TM

As indicated by Mankoff et al. (2004), there are three major obstacles to effective TM in practice. The first is the challenge of translating basic science discoveries into clinical studies. The second hurdle is the translation of clinical studies into medical practice and healthcare policy. A third obstacle to effective TM is philosophical. It may be a mistake to think that basic science (without observations from the clinic and without epidemiological findings of possible associations between different diseases) will efficiently produce the novel therapies for human testing. Pilot studies, such as nonhuman and nonclinical studies, are often used to transition therapies developed using animal models to a clinical setting. Statisticians often assist in the planning and analysis of pilot studies. The purpose of this book is to provide a comprehensive review of the statistical design and methodology that are commonly employed in translational research.

1.5 Potential Impact of TM on R&D

The proposed TM approach would change the environment that currently exists, which aims to optimize each process, while providing minimal effort to completely integrate these processes. In many companies, management continually preaches for every contributing discipline to reach its highest point of excellence. We find excellence committees, centers of excellence, stretch goals, excellence goals, etc., existing in one form or the other, across numerous disciplines within many pharmaceutical companies. Yet, inadvertently, without a clear focus on integration, this may foster divisions within a company and serve to discourage communication and information exchange between disciplines. At best, the link between technical excellence and knowledge sharing is a weak one. It is not uncommon to find many preclinical scientists chanting a mantra of "animal studies cannot predict human results" and wandering on to run scientifically interesting studies that may not contribute to the critical path for the development of a drug. This is not to declare that such studies should not be run, but a concept of prioritization of those studies versus studies affecting critical path issues (e.g., dosing, efficacy, safety, etc.) can be made and the timing of the "nice to know" studies can be altered. Furthermore, a mindset of preclinical studies having limited value to human studies creates a huge schism between preclinical and clinical scientists. Within a TM paradigm, excellence, though still recognized as a personal goal, is viewed on a different level than the requirement of transferring that knowledge across disciplines. Integration is a much clearer goal in a TM approach. Furthermore, concise high-level goals (e.g., put valuable drugs on the market, learn all we can about this drug, etc.) are shared across all disciplines. It does not focus on the number of publications, awards, citations, presentations, or any other personal indicators of achievement, all pleasant but not critical, but instead, gauges the value of activities in terms of how they impact on the common high-level goals. Thus, activities like integration are highly valued and encouraged. TM also challenges the attitude of limited extrapolation of animal data. Instead, it offers a viewpoint that there always remains a positive existence of some level of correlation (translation) between any particular outcome in an appropriate animal model and humans. The identification or quantification of this relationship in all cases is uncertain, but unless the two processes are strictly random, which is quite rare, some link function certainly exists. Furthermore, the TM approach stresses joint responsibility among all scientists in all phases of R&D, for all the decision making that is made during the entire R&D process.

Details of how a TM approach would impact the key processes and strategies for extracting potential benefit from such changes are discussed in Chapter 2. As mentioned, Chapter 3 presents a detailed discussion of a variety of data types and experiments carried out in a productive biomarker laboratory, followed by a discussion of the optimal statistical methods for each of the specified experiments. Chapter 4 continues with the discussion on the biomarker development. Chapter 5 brings more details on the targeted clinical studies employing TM methods, and Chapter 6 concentrates on some specialized statistical methods developed for studies where translational information is a key target of the study. Chapter 7 introduces the nonparametric approaches to the analysis of data from these translational studies, and Chapter 8 presents an approach for building, executing, and validating statistical models that consider data from various phases of development. Chapter 9 focuses on bridging studies that target clarification of relationships between numerous study endpoints, while Chapter 10 introduces a truly "translational" example when we take a look at finding links between traditional Chinese medicine's empirically based approaches existing for 5000 years and the experiment-based approaches employed in Western medicine.

For each chapter, real examples are given to illustrate the concepts, application, and limitations of statistical methods and potential value in adapting TM approaches. Wherever applicable, topics for possible further discussion or future research development are provided.

References

Mankoff, S.P., Brander, C., Ferrone, S., and Marincola, F.M., 2004. Lost in translation: obstacles to translational medicine. *Journal of Translational Medicine*, 2, 14.

Owens, J., 2007. 2006 drug approvals: finding the niche. *Nat. Drug Discov.*, 6, 99.

Chapter 2

Strategic Concepts in Translational Medicine

Dennis Cosmatos, Giora Feuerstein, and Shein-Chung Chow

Contents

It is important to recognize drug development as a decision-based science. Current evidence suggests that this recognition is not yet in place as inadequate consideration is placed on the consequences of wrong decisions in any part of the process, and that any such wrong decision will contribute to the failure rate. Evidence for this oversight is illustrated by examining the resource distribution in any pharmaceutical company, academic laboratory, or research division. Data gathering, as a generic term for the design, execution and collection, as well as storing of data in a given experiment, is the focus of most of the scientific research. Furthermore, planning, funding, personnel, and even visibility focus on these activities. Then, what proportion of time is spent conducting these data gathering activities versus the time spent conducting the analysis and performing a careful synthesis of the information? How carefully are decisions made from the data scrutinized and discussed among scientists before a final decision is taken? In almost all the research settings, it is obvious that this is the last, most hurried, and least collaborative activity. In many research settings, the individual best trained to perform the analyses, the statistician, is not even involved. This is especially, and perhaps unitarily, true in the early stage of research. For some reason, error in these early stages is tolerated, even expected. Then, when the paradigm shifts and the experiments are carried out for registration purposes (phase III clinical studies bound for registration/submission), the team would be ready to put more serious effort into analysis, to ensure correct decision making. In some sense, they are forced by regulatory agencies to ensure that they make correct decisions, and statisticians suddenly find themselves consulted on the study design, monitoring, and final analysis as predefined by an approved analysis plan. This gives rise to the following questions: Are the experiments carried out early in the R&D process that impact compound selection, dose selection, safety assessment, or preclinical efficacy any less important? Is error in the decision making more tolerable in these early stages? Is the magnitude of such error smaller in these early stages? Do most of today's research organizations quantify the level of error or manage it to be the customary 5% Type I and 20% Type II levels typical in the late stage research? Is there any consideration given to the presence of such errors in these early stages? Are optimal scientific designs being implemented in these early phases? Unfortunately, for the majority of pharmaceutical companies as well as academic laboratories, the answers to all the above questions are negative. It is our personal belief that this is a significant contributor to the high failure rate we observe under the current processes.

What we offer for consideration is a translational medicine (TM) decision-making mindset, resulting in radical changes in the way research is conducted and decisions are made in the early and late stages, not only in the pharmaceutical sector, but in all scientific sectors. The strong presence of statistical thinking in TM will evolve this discipline into one that will improve the "correctness" of all data-based decisions made within a given decision-driven process. With increased inter-disciplinary collaboration in decision making, a broader range of information will be considered for every decision. Proper experimental designs, focused decision steps, and proper analyses carried out within a TM structure will yield higher success rates and ultimately higher quality outcomes (drugs, biologics, etc.) in all types of research that adopt this paradigm. Improved decision making will also be assisted by the implementation of biomarkers. A key contribution of TM is the focused role of discovering, validating, and implementing biomarkers that can serve in lieu of clinical outcomes and accelerate the testing of efficacy or safety of a compound. Figure 2.1 illustrates how TM positions itself between discovery and clinical development, organized by therapeutic areas being investigated by the company. Its impact and activities begin as early as discovery and continues through phase III. An overview of how it interacts within each phase of R&D is detailed below.

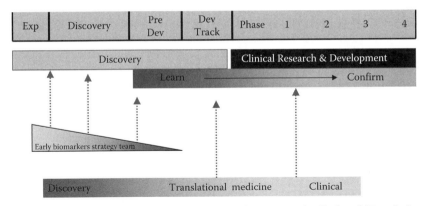

FIGURE 2.1: Role of TM in R&D. (From G. Feuerstein, Role of Translational Medicine across Research & Development. Original presentation slide, 2007.)

2.1 TM Approaches in Pharmaceutical Development

It is well known that pharmaceutical development is a lengthy and costly process. In addition, whatever process is followed, it must assure that the approved drug product will possess good drug characteristics, such as safety, identity, purity, quality, strength, stability, and reproducibility. A typical pharmaceutical development process involves drug discovery, formulation, laboratory development, animal studies for safety and efficacy estimation, clinical development, and regulatory submission/review and approval. In some organizations, a concept of Learn and Confirm define the R&D process with all early development, clinical and preclinical studies, and early clinical studies under the Learn phase. Only after adequately learning about the drug and its effects, would the compounds enter a Confirm phase where registration phase III studies are conducted. TM spans these two large development phases and even extends further into discovery.

For our discussion, we will concentrate on the more generic breakdown of the R&D process by defining three distinct research phases:

1. Nonclinical development (e.g., drug discovery, formulation, laboratory development, scale-up, manufacturing process validation, stability, and quality control/assurance)—chemists and biologists involved.

2. Preclinical development (e.g., animal studies for toxicity, bioavailability and bioequivalence studies, pharmacokinetic studies, and pharmacodynamic studies estimating potential efficacy)—biologists and veterinarians are the key contributors.

3. Clinical development (e.g., phases I–III clinical trials for assessment of safety and efficacy)—clinicians, clinical scientists, data managers, regulatory specialists, statisticians, and statistical programmers are involved.

These phases may occur in sequential order or may be somewhat overlapping during the development process. Key decision-making activities within these critical phases of pharmaceutical development are detailed below along with a discussion of how a TM strategy would impact on the behavior of those activities and what the possible benefit of such an approach would be. Admittedly, there is some oversimplification of this highly technical and complex set of activities. However, we try to capture the major points that can be influenced by the process changes and strategies suggested by adopting a TM approach.

2.1.1   Nonclinical Development

Nonclinical development includes drug discovery, formulation, laboratory development, such as analytical method development and validation, (manufacturing) process validation, stability, statistical quality control, and quality assurance (see, e.g., Chow and Liu, 1995).

2.1.1.1   Drug Discovery

Drug discovery is one of the first steps in the R&D process. At the drug-screening phase, numerous compounds are screened to identify those that are active from those that are not. Numerous *in vitro* experiments are carried out and a singular value, like an IC_{50} or LD_{50}, usually a mean of values across 3–6 replicates, is derived for each compound and is the key in the decision to select one compound over another to undergo further development as the lead compound, first backup, second backup, etc., or to be discarded. This is one of the first critical paths for the decisions to be made, and thus, the first opportunity to make a correct or incorrect decision.

However, drug potency is not the only decision-making statistic considered in compound selection. Characteristics of the drug with respect to the potential for inducing negative cardiac effects (HERG Channel Assay), its affinity to the intended target, and its biodistribution to intended and unintended biologic targets are all additional assessments made and considered in the selection process. These assay results are also important in dose selection (Section 2.2).

Current organizational structures make these decisions in a somewhat confined manner within the discipline of laboratory chemistry with some input from biologists. However, the belief exists that excellence in these disciplines will result in excellence in this critical decision making. As stated earlier, implementation of a TM approach would demand this level of expertise, yet further focus on having these individuals as a part of a multidisciplinary group would result in decisions based on full knowledge from individuals from many other disciplines. These individuals from other disciplines may have a deep understanding of the target population for the drug being considered, the market placement, and its relative value to the patient or caregiver. Further, statistical input would contribute to more robust examination of the data.

Empirically, the statistical point to be made is that the current decision process focuses on several point estimates (e.g., mean values of bioavailability measures, target occupancy estimates, IC_{50}, or LD_{50}). Statistical input would require not only the means of these measures, but also the individual values to be considered and reported (min, max, median, and standard deviation across the experiments for each compound). Then, with the given observed level of variability across the individual assays, a sample size sensitive to the level of variability and computed under acceptable levels of Type I and Type II error can be computed and, when needed, additional assays can be carried out to provide more reliable estimates of these important decision-making measures. Alternatively, strong consideration would be given to those compounds with lower variability in one or more of these measures, rather than the highest value (e.g., potency measures). For example, for a particular formulation, the potency can be improved by increasing the dose, but high variability cannot be addressed that easily and will impact on all the decisions being made as the compound proceeds through development (more detailed discussion is given later in Section 2.1.3). Unfortunately, at this stage, we may have limited information on whether the dose can be escalated, as initial *in vivo* toxicology studies might not have been carried out. In a proper TM approach, this is a point we can come back to, if further development suggests that we can produce higher doses and there is adequate safety for higher doses. This flexibility may induce some increased costs or time delays, but this needs to be balanced against the "cost" of ignoring variability observed in these very controlled experiments, and continuing with a compound that might have even greater variability in animal and human systems. Repeatedly, such compounds yield difficult estimation properties and perhaps are more prone to failure at a later stage after additional resources are invested.

2.1.1.2 Formulation

The purpose of formulation is to develop a dosage form (e.g., tablets or capsules) such that the drug can be delivered to the site of action efficiently. Oftentimes, a lead candidate identified in drug discovery can be modified to have better dosing properties by making changes in the formulation of the compound. This may involve using alternative dissolution solvents, substrates to carry the active drug, coatings to adjust dose release, etc. In this multifactorial setting, statistical input and close collaboration with TM associates could influence many aspects of the designs of experiments carried out to optimize the formulation. Input from marketing and clinical can prioritize the importance of properties like need for slow release, need for higher dose strengths, etc. Again, most importantly, this needs to be a function that we can return to after having some preclinical or clinical experience with the drug. A TM strategy would encourage this, where, currently, returning to formulation is a reluctant practice and sometimes, the available dosage forms affects the important dose decisions. From a distance, this may seem like a case of "the tail wagging the dog," yet it is surprising as to how many times a drug development program is stalled or permanently impeded, because too many of the capsules or tablets produced would be needed to hit the target dose. Or conversely, additional safety with equivalent efficacy could be gained with a slightly lower dose that is not available from current formulation.

2.1.1.3   Laboratory Development/Validation/Analytic Methods

For laboratory development, an analytical method is necessarily developed to quantitate the potency (strength) of the drug product. Analytical method development and validation plays an important role in quality control and quality assurance of the drug product. To ensure that a drug product will meet the USP/NF (2000) standards for the identity, strength, quality, and purity of the drug product, a number of tests, such as potency testing, weight variation testing, content uniformity testing, dissolution testing, and disintegration testing are usually performed at various stages of the manufacturing process. These tests are referred to as USP/NF tests.

Important consideration needs to be given in the measurement error in the developed assays. All too often, we accept drug assays with 15% level of error or higher. For some reason, this has been deemed acceptable. This contributes to having observed drug concentrations as measured by values like C_{max} and AUC having a 30% CV or more, among the subjects. This can lead to observing a 15% level of response in an exposure–response model as very unreliable. Again, this level of error contributes to the wrong decisions in dose selection currently being made.

2.1.1.4   Manufacturing Process Validation

After the drug product has been approved by the regulatory agency for use in humans, a scale-up program is usually carried out to ensure that a production batch can meet USP/NF standards for the identity, strength, quality, and purity of the drug before a batch of the product is released to the market. The purpose of a scale-up program is not only to identify, evaluate, and optimize critical formulation or (manufacturing) process factors of the drug product, but also to maximize or minimize recipient range. A successful scale-up program can result in an improvement in the formulation/process or at least a recommendation on a revised procedure for formulation/process of the drug product. During the nonclinical development, the manufacturing process is necessarily validated to produce drug products with good drug characteristics, such as identity, purity, strength, quality, stability, and reproducibility. Process validation is important in nonclinical development to ensure that the manufacturing process does what it purports to do. The difficulty exists in scaling up the production of pills having set doses when the dose selection process is still not completed, which is often the case. Yet another reason why accuracy and expediency of dose selection are of high importance to the R&D process.

2.1.1.5   Stability, Drug Substance Quality Control, and Quality Assurance

Stability studies are usually conducted to characterize the degradation of the drug product over time, under appropriate storage condition. Stability data can then be used to determine drug expiry-date period (or drug shelf life), required by the regulatory agency to be indicated in the immediate label of the container. Again, the need for finalization of the dose decision impacts on when these studies can start as the stability needs to be determined on a given formulation, in a given form (capsule or tablet), and at a given dose.

2.1.2 Preclinical Development

Preclinical development evaluates the safety and efficacy of drug products through *in vitro* assays and animal studies. In general, *in vitro* assays or animal toxicity studies are intended to alert the clinical investigators to the potential toxic effects associated with the investigated drugs so that those effects may be looked out for during the clinical investigation. Preclinical testing sets the groundwork for dose selection, toxicological testing for toxicity and carcinogenicity, and animal pharmacokinetics. For selection of an appropriate dose, dose-response (dose ranging) studies in animals are usually conducted to determine the effective dose, such as the median effective dose (ED_{50}). Preclinical development is critical in pharmaceutical development process, because it is not ethical to investigate certain toxicities, such as the impairment of fertility, teratology, mutagenicity, and overdose in humans (Chow and Liu, 1998). Animal models are then used as a surrogate for human testing under the assumption that they can be predictive of the clinical outcomes in humans.

The acronym ADME—absorption, distribution, metabolism, and excretion—accurately summarizes the type of information gained from these early animal studies. In addition, the later animal studies looking at pharmacodynamic (i.e., efficacy) outcomes are the key in determining the future of the drug. Dose selection, dose regimen, and safe dose levels are parameters that are all joined to results observed in this stage. A poor safety profile, "drugability" profile, or efficacy profile at this stage will certainly doom the success of the drug in further development. Given this, one would think that the greatest level of precision and care in making correct decisions should be applied at this phase of development. For a proper "translation" to occur, a TM approach also requires accuracy in these data. In the subsequent discussion, we will highlight the fact that the most significant changes needed to improve the success rate in drug development are required at this phase. In addition, as mentioned, biologists and veterinarians are key contributors and in some companies sole contributors to the design, execution, and conclusions drawn from studies conducted in this phase. Expanding this group to include many more scientists and disciplines is the cornerstone of creating an effective TM strategy and gaining true benefit from such a strategy. The result may be in terminating more drugs at this stage that may pose some challenges in meeting some company metrics. However, we believe that the advantages in saving development costs and having an improved success rate will be much more beneficial than simply meeting a metric.

2.1.2.1 Preclinical Safety

The animal safety studies that must be conducted to clear a drug for use in humans are well documented in FDA and ICH Guidances (Arcy and Harron, 1992; FDA, 1996; ICH Harmonised Tripartite Guidelines (S1A, S2A, S3A, S5A, and S5B); ICH Topic S2B Document; ICH Topic S4 Document; ICH Topic S6 Document). The overriding caveat for animal studies is: "Studies should be designed so that the maximum amount of information is obtained from the smallest number of animals" as quoted from an FDA/ICH Guidance. This goes well with most pharmaceutical companies, as this also translates to quicker and less expensive investment at this phase. However, an accompanying caveat should raise the issue of unethical use of animal resources when studies are carried out that are not adequately powered to answer proper scientific questions. In a clinical setting, an IRB (institutional review board) would/should not approve a clinical study that is underpowered to answer the primary clinical questions, and consequently, we should hold the same test to our animal studies to assure the ethical use of animals.

In most R&D programs, the first animal study to be carried out with a new drug is typically an escalating dose study, characteristically in rats (sometimes mice), with dose levels in milligram per kilogram, escalating to 10-fold or more, with three dose levels. Again, this is typical, but there are some variations according to drug properties identified in the nonclinical phase. For example, a 14-day rat safety study may dose three animals at each of three dose levels: 10, 100, and 1000 mg/kg, a total of nine animals. This study is also repeated in a nonrodent mammal with even fewer animals per dose group. Most often, if toxicities are observed, they are observed at the dose of 1000 mg/kg, and 100 mg/kg receives the important designation of the NOAEL (no observable adverse effect level). The resulting drug concentrations of animals dosed at that level are also noted.

As dose selection continues, depending on the targeted drug indication and observed toxicities seen in the animal models, scaled human doses will be influenced by the identified NOAEL. For severe illnesses, the maximum human dose allowed for testing may be near the NOAEL or even slightly above. However, for nonlethal diseases, the tolerance is much lower and drug concentrations near 1/10th of those seen in the NOAEL dose serve as the maximum.

Several questions arise when such a design is implemented. First, "what is the safety profile between 100 mg/kg and 1000 mg/kg? When optimizing dose and, more importantly, exposure in humans, do we currently have enough information with such a small study? What conclusion do we draw when drug concentrations vary widely, perhaps across dosing groups? How accurately are safety levels evaluated in animal models like the beagle dog, where emesis, a common defense mechanism in these dogs, results in much of the drug not being ingested? Occasionally, some more definitions will be requested when efficacy (human or animal) is not seen at the highest dose tested and more information is requested (i.e., more animal studies are carried out), but this is very rare. More frequently, development of that compound is terminated for "lack of efficacy." Again, this is a situation that may have possible decision error contributing to the overall low success rate.

A TM approach would greatly impact in this context as a back-and-forth discussion and assignment of tasks takes place and is even expected. Especially, after the first clinical dose is administered, a detailed "translation" can be made between drug concentrations seen in humans versus all the animal models. We can then better assess where we are on the safety/efficacy curve. If there is need for more information from animals, the resources are there to go back and "clear" higher dose, perhaps doses between the 100 mg/kg and 1000 mg/kg range.

2.1.2.2 Bioavailability, Bioequivalence, and Animal Pharmacokinetic Studies

Following the administration of a drug, it is important to study the rate and extent of absorption, the amount of drug in the bloodstream consequently becoming available, and the elimination of the drug. For this purpose, a comparative bioavailability study in humans is usually conducted to characterize the profile of the blood or plasma concentration–time curve by means of several pharmacokinetic parameters, such as area under the blood or plasma concentration–time curve (AUC), maximum concentration (C_{max}), and time to achieve maximum concentration (t_{max}) (Chow and Liu, 2000). It should be noted that the identified compounds will have to pass the stages of nonclinical/preclinical development before they can be used in humans. As many aspects of the drug are easier to test in animals than in humans, it is especially reasonable to assume that even though the dosing of a drug will be adjusted from animals to a human, the relative effects between doses may carry over quite well. For example, the relationship between dose and drug availability as measured either by pharmacokinetic measures in the animal or using receptor occupancy measures using some imaging tools, may carry over quite well between animals and humans. Although the overall bioavailability varies with the animal species, this relationship with dose may carry over across the animal species and even translate well into the human model.

One aspect to consider is trying to obtain more information from these animal models by running them using designs like crossover, allowing exposure of a single animal to more than one dose group. This will allow better estimates for dose proportionality and ADME assessment within an animal. Obviously, this can be done only when adequate washout of the drug is possible. This design can also be especially useful when examining biodistribution or receptor occupancy.

There are some technological requirements that need to be developed that will substantially improve our measurement of drug availability and concentration in animal models. One in particular is the use of a micro-dosing assay for assessing drug concentrations in an animal. Presently, the amount of blood needed for accurately assessing drug concentration affects the animal's performance and even viability, and hence, repeat dosing is not possible. The development of a micro-dosing assay that can measure these levels at lower doses will be the key in allowing the proper interpretation of dose ranges (see more discussion on dose selection in Section 2.2).

Once the drug is tested in humans, then all the relating information gathered in the animal models is made much clearer. A TM approach would dedicate more time in making this link, refining allometric models that predict human dose ranges and reexamine safety findings given in this critical translation key (again, there will be more discussion on this under dose selection in Section 2.2).

2.1.2.3 Animal Pharmacodynamic Studies

As mentioned earlier, animal pharmacodynamic studies are the key studies in the pharmaceutical R&D process. Admittedly, the safety and ADME studies often are primary "killers" or no-go generators. However, the tone turns in this phase of development. Rather than looking for a reason to "kill" a drug and being liberal with our acceptance of Type I error (as it would allow us to be more conservative), we now seek reasons for further investment into development of a drug candidate. Although not often admitted, experience has shown that failure to see some hint of efficacy at this phase will almost surely halt the development of any drug.

The obvious challenge is that human diseases are not always observed in animals. Hence, frequently, animal models are developed to either mimic certain aspects of a disease (e.g., cognition, memory, and attentiveness as symptoms affected by diseases like Alzheimer's disease and schizophrenia), or created to focus on the biologic target that the drug is affecting. For example, when a particular biologic target is identified as being critical in a disease pathway, knockout (KO) animals can be created that allow us to see what the maximum effect of suppressing that target can suggest or allow us to observe specific effects of our drugs on those animals. In some therapeutic areas (e.g., asthma, hypercholesterolemia, diabetes), a disease model is available and the effect of our drug on animals with that specific disease can be used to directly test the efficacy of the test compound on that disease.

As these are critical experiments, one would think that they would be receiving the same level of resources and review as the compatible clinical studies. Yet, across the industry and in many academic laboratories, we routinely observe underpowered, poorly designed, and poorly analyzed animal efficacy studies. In a situation where it would require a large phase III clinical study to observe drug effect on a given disease, there is some underlying logic that assumes that same level of efficacy can be observed in a small animal experiment with 10 or 20 animals. Rarely, if ever, do the animal studies quote a level of power justifying the sample size used.

A TM approach would directly challenge this mindset. Gathering initial efficacy information like drug concentration, target occupancy, or establishing initial dose–response estimates in a small study is acceptable, as long as it is followed up by a scientifically valid, properly powered decision-making study. The commonly identified "minimally efficacious dose" (MED) should be replaced with a well-defined exposure–response curve looking at changes in the efficacy with changes in the dose/concentration. Establishing concentration levels at the observed levels of efficacy is itself an issue, as the blood draws needed to derive drug concentrations would impact the animal's performance on any efficacy measure, when using small animals. Here again, there is a need for the development of a micro-dosing assay capable of substantially reducing the blood volume needed to establish drug concentration levels, where possible crossover designs would also benefit our understanding of the drug effect. Also, the inclusion of an active control in the study design is often overlooked. Even if the active control has an effect using an alternative mechanism of action than the test drug, it is of value to quantify how the test drug can be compared with the existing treatments for a given disease. Overall, statistical input into each and every animal efficacy study should be mandated to ensure that correct decisions are made from the results of these studies. In this setting, a Type II error can be more costly than a Type I error, as incorrectly passing up a truly safe and efficacious drug, after the investment already made to prove its safety, wastes substantial company resources and impacts on the overall success rate and value linked with the company by outside investors. A phase I error is very likely to be picked up in the early clinical studies.

2.1.3 Clinical Development

Clinical development of a pharmaceutical entity is to scientifically evaluate benefits (e.g., efficacy) and risks (e.g., safety) of promising pharmaceutical entities in humans at a minimum cost and time frame. The impact of TM will be greatest at this juncture, where information from the prior nonclinical and preclinical phases is used to design informative and decisive clinical studies. It should be appreciated at this juncture that the success of the clinical studies is directly linked with the successful development of a compound through these earlier trials in animals and on the laboratory bench. Ownership and understanding of these earlier studies, jointly by the clinical scientists and the research scientists is the core of a TM strategy. This is not, as currently, a "deliverable" to clinical and a hands-off approach from early research scientists. This current strategy has led to the "finger-pointing" that currently occurs when questioning the reasons for a poor success rate. The clinical scientists may claim that the compounds handed to them were not well identified and formulated, and the research scientists may claim that the clinical trials were carried without understanding and proper use of the compounds they passed down, and that they cannot be held responsible for the species differences inherent in them. More discussion on this issue can be observed in Section 2.2, where an approach to changing this mindset is suggested and is embedded in the dose-selection process.

2.1.3.1 First-in-Human (Phase I) Studies

The primary objective of phase I studies is not only to determine the metabolism and pharmacological activities of the drug in humans, the side effects associated with increasing doses, and the early evidence on effectiveness, but also to obtain sufficient information about the drug's pharmacokinetics and pharmacological effects to permit the design of well-controlled and scientifically valid phase II studies. First-in-human studies provide an extraordinary opportunity to integrate (translate) information from basic research, such as pharmacokinetics, pharmacodynamics, and toxicology while launching the new molecule on a path for rational clinical development in humans. Traditionally, basic research has been separated from the clinical practice of medicine without much communication. As a result, much information obtained about a drug in the preclinical stages is lost or ignored. This process is not only inefficient, but also decreases the probability of success in pharmaceutical development.

Typical designs for an FIH study in most therapeutic areas (excluding oncology) involves selection of 5–7 dose levels and introducing 8 healthy volunteers at each dose level, escalating through all the dose levels unless a safety signal prevents advancement. Of the eight volunteers, six are randomized to receive a designated dose of the drug and two receive a placebo, often disguised to look like the test product. This sample size is often justified by arguments that with this number of treated subjects we can adequate power to observe adverse events with fairly high levels of occurrence.

... six subjects [receiving the test drug] in each cohort provides 47%, 62%, 74%, or 82% probability of observing at least one occurrence of any adverse event, when the true incidence rate for a given dose cohort is 10%, 15%, 20%, or 25%, respectively ...

This is a set design used for most of the drugs in all nononcologic therapeutic areas. It may be possible that all compounds entering this phase of development may not have the same underlying characteristics, with varying absorption profiles, different distributional properties, perhaps varying levels of exposure at a given dose, etc. So, if the design is the same and the compounds differ, it can be concluded that what reflects those differences is in the quality of the conclusions made from these studies, before even addressing how decisions on dose ranges are made. To illustrate, consider one compound with the typical 30% CV in key pharmacokinetic parameter estimates (e.g., C_{max} or AUC_{0-Inf}) against an alternative compound with 70% CV. When assessing drug concentrations, using this set $6 + 2$ design, our estimates for the first compound will have better precision than that of the second compound. We will be able to get point estimates in the forms of means or medians for both compounds, but owing to having a fixed sample size, the variability around those estimates will be greater for the compound with the greater CV. Unfortunately, the conclusions drawn and determinations on safety and pharmacokinetic properties rarely consider this difference in precision and would often treat estimates from both such compounds as being equally reliable when passing on dose recommendations to the phase II studies.

An alternative strategy would be suggested by a TM approach. A study design could be considered where appreciation for the compound properties would be used in an adaptive manner to modify the study as it progresses, and maintain a constant level of precision from all the pharmacokinetic and pharmacologic estimates derived from the study. First, the initial dose would enter the typical $6 + 2$ healthy volunteers. An examination upon completion of this first dose would yield initial estimates on variability of these key pharmacokinetic parameter estimates and compute the sample size needed at that particular dose level to maintain a given, say 20%, level of precision around these estimates. If the sample size is 6, then no adjustment is made, if the sample size is $6 + n^*$, then the n^* subjects would be entered when the next dose group is opened for accrual. This second dose group could assume that the variability is the same as the first and begin accruing $6 + n^*$ active subjects for the study with the second dose. Another evaluation could be made after completion of the second dose group to observe if the level of precision is met for the first and second dose group. As we often observe increasing variability with increasing dose, it is quite likely that additional subjects ($6 + n^* + m^*$) would be needed at the second dose level to maintain the stated level of precision. Then, those m^* number of subjects would be entered in the third dose group. If not, the study could continue with $6 + n^*$ subjects for the subsequent dose groups, rechecking after each is completed.

Alternatively, animal data can provide some warning of highly variable absorption or metabolism of a compound. In those cases, we should probably start with a larger sample size, about 8–10 to begin with. Then, after some data, we can check its correlation with the animal results and see if subsequent PK characteristics in higher doses continue to have this trend. More formally, we can examine how to translate the animal result to human and proceed in a much more knowledgeable manner. Even if absolute drug-concentration profiles differ drastically between animals and humans, typically owing to differing metabolisms, the relative changes in these characteristics across dose levels may in fact be well predicted by the animal studies.

As the most intensive drug information is obtained in these early clinical studies, resources to investigate precise exposure–response and exposure–safety relationships should be dedicated to every study. Other studies conducted in this phase (e.g., drug interaction, hepatic impairment, QTc studies, etc.) also provide us insight into the way a particular drug behaves in humans. Yet, the ominous timeline for development often curtails the thoroughness of analyses in this stage and forces short and quick studies to be the targeted behavior. In Section 2.2, we will see how a TM structure involved at this stage could change this type of behavior. Also, in Section 2.3 we will see how the mergence of biomarkers has given even further importance to these early studies in supplying early evidence of drug activity or mechanism of action evidence.

Another study design to consider is a "rotating panel" design where a singe dose is administered to a given healthy human volunteer, and after adequate washout, that individual can return to receive another dosing of whatever dose level is open for accrual. This design will offer valuable within-subject drug information, and even if this is available for just a few subjects, it can be used to compare with what was observed in the animals, which again makes this prior information quite valuable in better understanding of dose proportionality, absorption profile, early evidence of dose accumulation effects, and much more information. Obviously, this design is limited to those compounds having short half-lives and acceptable safety. The only concern voiced over such a design is the decrease in the number of individuals exposed to the drug, and thus, estimate of safety assessment. Yet, one could argue that the early repeated dosing contributes to our detection of certain types of drug-induced safety concerns.

Early clinical studies subsequently advance into multiple, ascending dose studies. Again, the set 6 + 2 design is often used in these studies. Amazingly, this design is pursued even after initial single-dose studies demonstrate high variability in pharmacokinetic measures at some or all of the administered doses. A TM approach would consider making the adjustments in the sample size of each dose level, as suggested earlier, fixing the level of desired precision for each pharmacokinetic parameter to be estimated.

Perhaps the highest visibility of TM in these early stages is the introduction of biomarkers into these early studies. Often little validation of these biomarkers in human applications has been conducted at this point and hence, these studies can provide this information and help prepare the use of these biomarkers as decision tools in later studies. In a few instances, TM scientists have indeed completed validation of these biomarkers in a given disease pathway, and understanding about how the drug affects this pathway can be obtained in these early studies. Subsequently, adjustments in dose or regimen can be considered as the final dose selection is made.

2.1.3.2   Phase II Studies

The primary objectives of phase II studies are not only to first evaluate the effectiveness of a drug based on clinical endpoints for a particular indications in patients with the disease or condition under study, but also to determine the dosing ranges and doses for phase III studies and the common short-term side effects and risks associated with the drug. TM still has a major presence in this phase as it continues to provide learned information from the earlier stages.

2.1.3.3   Phase III Studies

The primary objectives of phase III studies are to (1) gather additional information about the effectiveness and safety needed to evaluate the overall benefit–risk relationship of the drug and (2) to provide an adequate basis for physician labeling. The studies in this phase of development serve to form the key submission documents reviewed by a regulatory agency before a drug is approved for marketing in the country or countries governed by that agency. A failure to file or rejection of approval at this stage is the most serious event a company can face and is almost immediately reflected by the investor community, resulting in a reduction in the stock price of that company, if it is publicly held. Yet, as mentioned in Section 2.1.2, the rate of failure at this phase in 2003 reached as high as 50% and this was most often owing to the sponsor selecting the incorrect dose or regimen for these pivotal studies, resulting in unacceptable toxicities or low evidence of efficacy. We should view this as a culmination of all prior researches leading to this incorrect decision to conduct these critical studies at the selected doses. More broadly, poor understanding of the true exposure–response of our drugs is the key in causing this critical misjudgment. TM will soon be considered as a key discipline that prevents this type of error and provides the greatest volume of information concerning all characteristics: safety, efficacy, and variability of these outcomes in a heterogeneous population and in special populations, of a given drug. In the following section, we will discuss how TM can carry out this, beginning with a TM approach to dose selection.

2.2   TM Approaches to Dose Selection

It is unchallenged that dose selection is one of the most important decisions to be made in the clinical development process. Yet, across companies, there is no consistent or detailed process specified on how this important decision is reached. Sometimes, it is reached by a small collection of clinical scientists soon after phase II, while at times it is reached by a broader set of clinical and basic scientists, formally or informally. Yet, we must recognize that it a decision that is impacted by the very first discovery scientist who conducts the initial *in vitro* study, examining the early efficacy on a cell culture. It is then refined as the process continues, but at every step, its fate is influenced, often without being carefully recognized by the action of a single scientist. Within this section, we propose a well-defined process for taking careful consideration, careful actions, and careful cross-disciplinary decisions when making this determination at each step of the development process. A set of four critical face-to-face meetings of all scientists involved is suggested and defined in the following section.

2.2.1 Dose Selection Prior to Phase I: Meeting 1

This will be the largest, most broadly attended, and likely to be the longest duration of the four meetings. Careful consideration is taken for every preclinical experiment conducted to date, including the early discovery findings and establishment of LD_{50} or ED_{50} values, early toxicology findings, early animal ADME findings, and early animal efficacy findings. Attendees of this meeting should include:

- Translational scientists to evaluate "translation ability" of the data and relate past knowledge on this from prior similar compounds examined. (cochair)

- Statisticians to ensure that accurate study designs and data analyses were performed across all prior studies. (cochair)

- Discovery scientists to review *in vitro* data

- Preclinical scientists to review animal efficacy data

- Toxicologists to discuss animal safety results to date

- ADME scientists to discuss animal pharmacokinetic findings

- Formulation specialists to discuss production options

- Production-plant scientists to assess drug quality/quantity issues

- Clinical pharmacologists to design first-in-human studies and clinical plan

- Clinical pharmacokineticists to help plan the future clinical PK studies, review animal PK data, and contribute to the allometric scaling effort

- Marketing representatives to discuss market focus for the drug and target product profiles

At this meeting some critical decisions made in earlier step are reviewed. Working as a TM Group, any challenges could and should arise in a collegial fashion with a willingness to fairly assess if a past step needs to be rerun either in the future or before the project can advance, depending on the importance of obtaining the modified information for that step. Critical evaluation of prior experiments that impart dose selection decisions (e.g., hERG channel assay, NOAEL dose, MED, etc.) are carefully reviewed with respect to the chances of avoiding an incorrect dose selection decision. Again, if further information is needed, it will need to be obtained with agreement over its timing and impact on moving forward. In the current paradigm, individual metrics for each of these groups (number of compounds brought to development, amount of time to complete animal toxicology, and ADME studies, etc.), impact on the quality and certainty of the information obtained.

A recurring statistical comment sure to be made is the avoidance of making any decisions based on a point estimate. All information concerning the variability of every point estimate needs to be reviewed. Sometimes, the estimate of variability rather than the point estimate itself may lead to a certain key decision. For example, if in animal studies, we observe a marked increase in the variability of pharmacokinetic properties of a drug when the drug reaches a certain level of exposure, then we may consider changing the dosing regimen (e.g., BID vs. QD) with a lesser dose or asking for some formulation changes to allow a slow release of the drug.

Results of any allometric scaling computations should be very closely examined at this meeting and fully critiqued. When possible, a "Physiologic" Allometric Scaling procedure should be employed. The "one size fits all" approach suggested in the FDA Guidance for Industry (FDA, 2002) should be carefully examined for appropriateness to the drug being developed. In this Guidance, a simple method to convert animal doses (in milligram per kilogram) to human doses (in mg assuming an average 60 kg human) is suggested:

$$HED = \text{animal dose} \times (\text{animal wt}/60)^{0.33}$$

Hence, for mouse, the animal dose must be divided by 12.3, rat dose by 6.2, rabbit by 3.1, dog by 1.8, etc. This formula is most influenced by known differences in animal size and metabolic rate. However, we know that there are so many other differences between animals and humans, such as metabolic enzymes, protein-binding mechanisms, immune mechanisms, etc., that the applicability of this simple conversion may be questionable for many new drugs as well as biologics. A physiologic model will attempt to correct many of these other factors affecting drug metabolism, drug–target affinity, and drug bioavailability.

The general question of translation between animal and human, especially as it relates to dosing, needs to be addressed separately with every drug. As TM asserts itself as a discipline, it will be invaluable in assembling this information across drugs and therapeutic areas and concentrate on establishing methods appropriate to perform this function more accurately. This is the reason for the suggestion of a cochair for this meeting. Statistics will also play a key role, as analyses across so many disciplines will be reviewed or conducted. Also, as mentioned, a quality check on decisions made versus data supporting those decisions will be driven by the statistician's evaluation of the data presented.

Apart from reviewing the past data, a significant part of the meeting is also spent in planning the upcoming clinical studies. An early clinical plan is drafted with input from the clinical scientists, clinical pharmacokineticists, and statisticians. In addition, input from marketing representatives can influence discussions on the drug characteristics (e.g., needs to be QD not BID) and allow discussion of appropriate competitor drugs on the market that can serve as active controls in our early studies.

Once again, the key aspect to the suggested paradigm is the ability to go back and perform a needed experiment to answer a critical question. It is of much greater value to the organization to increase the certainty and correctness of a dose decision, even at the cost of increasing the timeline, in that this decision directly impacts on the success rate of getting drugs to market.

While concluding this process, a firm decision is reached on the dose range that is to be investigated in the first human clinical trial. However, it must be expected that this range may be modified as the additional clinical studies are conducted.

2.2.2 Dose Selection Following the Initial First-in-Human Study: Meeting 2

In a rush to complete early clinical studies and advance the program to phases II and III, where it receives more recognition from the public and market analysts, adequate time to fully analyze, synthesize, and share early clinical results is often lacking. Yet, this first clinical study provides such a wealth of information that will allow us to link all preclinical findings with what is seen in humans. Our critical "link" between animal and clinical is obtained at this very first step into the clinical study. To fully assimilate all this information, the following people should attend a second meeting of the proposed Dose Selection Committee:

- Translational scientists who will be collecting information on "translation" between PK, exposure, safety, and efficacy (via biomarkers), observed in the clinical study with that seen in the animal experiments

- Statisticians to provide hands-on analyses supporting all translation activities and in-depth analyses of safety and dose– or exposure–response activity. (cochair)

- Discovery scientists to help in identifying such translation

- Preclinical scientists to evaluate animal efficacy data versus observed biomarker results, perhaps leading to another animal study

- Toxicologists to help identify safety patterns seen in both humans and animals

- ADME scientists to validate allometric scaling estimates and modify them if needed

- Formulation specialists to discuss production options that may be needed as the program proceeds, with respect to this early clinical PK data

- Production-plant scientists to assess drug quality/quantity issues

- Clinical pharmacologists to provide critical safety assessments and examine early information on drug tolerability

- Clinical pharmacokineticists to help plan future clinical PK studies, review animal PK data, and contribute to the allometric scaling effort (cochair)

This second meeting will focus on assessing how well earlier translation efforts worked and in making modifications based on the observed results. Most importantly, concentration information in animals can now be linked with the data on humans, and assessments on what dose may be beyond the NOAEL or maximum tolerated dose can be made. As much of the data from this first study is pharmacokinetic, the clinical pharmacokineticist serves as cochair of this meeting and ensures to obtain input from all other members. Again, activities prior to this meeting will rely heavily on the statistician to provide those TM analyses and clinical pharmacology analyses needed to glean most information from these data and build the TM knowledge base. To prepare for multiple dosing, an active discussion of all pharmacokinetic and safety data and its impact on the early clinical plans is reviewed with the team, led by the clinical pharmacologist. Outcomes suggesting possible drug–drug interaction (via CYP metabolism patterns) or cardiac risks (using EKG data) are reviewed. An evaluation of dose proportionality will also be made, which may have direct impact on the dose-escalation schedule to be followed.

If biomarkers were measured in the study, the translational scientists assess whether they are tracking any clinical endpoint or disease pathway, and discuss their possible interpretation and future use in subsequent clinical studies. Most valuable would be the identification of a biomarker that tracks the disease so well as to be considered as a candidate for development into a surrogate marker for the disease. This would provide great potential for accelerating the development program. If reasonable, the upcoming MAD study could be conducted in a patient population and the true utility of the biomarker can be assessed. In general, the opportunity to have the MAD study as a patient study should more often be considered, as the translation between healthy volunteers and patients can get very difficult when the disease in question imposes many physiologic changes. Safety, PK, and biomarker information may be quite different in patients than in healthy volunteers. If this is suspected, we need to design a clinical plan where we initiate patient studies as early as possible, even when the drug is still in the early development stage.

It is not rare that not only are many questions answered from this first study, but many new questions are also raised. Most notably, if we see unexpected drug pharmacokinetics, we need to reevaluate the path forward. Many times, however, we miss the opportunity to go back to animal studies to address such questions. Current company dynamics view development as a one-way street. Once the compound reaches humans, it is never to return to animal study. TM challenges this and notes that having the first human data provides us a link with the animal data, thus allowing us to design and execute meaningful and better-targeted animal studies. Cost is still less in conducting an animal experiment versus a human experiment and is likely to be quicker to provide an answer. Also, we would now be better in assessing the risk of linking this result from animal to human. A TM approach would encourage utilizing this valuable information and considering answering some new questions, if appropriate, back in an animal setting.

2.2.3 Dose Selection Prior to Phase II: Meeting 3

The early, phase I clinical program can range from an average of five studies to more than 20–30 studies before the compound advances to phase II, and continue with numerous formulation studies and special population studies, while the drug is proceeding through phases II and even phase III. Yet, there is a given point after key SAD and MAD studies that a decision is made to go into serious investment in the compound and begin phase II and III development. It is at this point that the third dose selection meeting is proposed. Attendees of this meeting would include:

- Translational scientists who will be leading discussions on what biomarkers are ready for further development or can provide key information on safety or efficacy

- Statisticians to ensure that all decisions are supported by adequate data and experiments and to plan the later development plan and provide needed analyses

- Preclinical scientists to evaluate animal efficacy data versus observed biomarker results, perhaps leading to another animal study

- Formulation specialists to discuss any needed changes in the drug product that may be needed as the program proceeds, with respect to this early clinical PK data

- Production-plant scientists to assess drug quality/quantity issues

- Clinical pharmacologists to provide critical safety assessments and examine early information on drug tolerability (cochair)

- Clinical pharmacokineticists to help plan future clinical PK studies, review animal PK data, and contribute to the allometric scaling effort (cochair)

- Clinical directors (MDs) involved in the later phase of the clinical program

- Marketing representatives to update on market competition and needed product profile

Often, the decision to go to phase II is fairly automatic, assuming adequate drug tolerability with the given intended treatment indication. This meeting is aimed at a thorough review of all early clinical data and objective decision making on what issues are still outstanding that may prevent successful registration of the test compound. The main issue, dose selection, becomes more critical as the options for modifying the dose range are narrowing. One approach is to enter phase II with a still broad range of doses and utilize an adaptive design (Chow and Chang, 2006) to select between these doses based on patient responses. This is in fact an appropriate option, but this should also signal a failure of the early activities to adequately characterize the drug. If translation efforts, biomarker information, pharmacokinetic studies, and pharmacodynamic studies were properly conducted, the only remaining question should be: Will there be adequate efficacy and acceptable drug tolerability in the patient population? The clinical pharmacologists and clinical pharmacokineticists cochair this meeting and lead the discussions on all these topics. Others in the meeting are critical in providing a link with the prior decisions made and in building the knowledge base that will extend across projects. TM scientists are still active participants, as much validation work needs to be performed on biomarkers when measured in a patient population (if the MAD studies were on healthy volunteers). Also, plans for obtaining and analyzing genomic, metabonomic, or proteomic data from the patient population are discussed. Imaging studies, possibly developed in healthy volunteers, are first applied to patients in phase II and can serve to provide a market advantage over a competitor drug that did not provide imaging evidence of efficacy. The marketing representative can provide input on how the marketplace has changed since initiation of the program and what, if any, new product characteristics are needed to remain competitive in the marketplace.

2.2.4   Dose Selection Prior to Phase III Registration Trials: Meeting 4

Assuming that the phase II studies have demonstrated adequate safety and efficacy in the patient population, the phase III studies should be strictly confirmatory. Proper dose selection for these trials is the most important decision to date. As before, incorrect information at any prior decision point will impact on the success of this study. A thorough review of all data and detailing of all decision points and resulting decisions should be presented to the medical team. Not only dose selection needs to be confirmed at this meeting, but discussion on other information to be collected is also discussed. These being the largest studies in a patient population, they provide the best opportunity for a TM scientist to conduct biomarker validation or gather adequate data for a meaningful genomic or proteomic analysis. This final meeting should contain the following people:

- Translational scientists who will be contributing the strategy for collection of biomarker data to either validate an existing biomarker or look for new genomic, metabonomic, and proteomic data that can enhance our understanding of the disease, mechanism of action of the drug, or provide data for new drug development (cochair).

- Statisticians have long been recognized as the key in the design of the pivotal studies and derivation of appropriate analysis plans that are to be submitted for regulatory review. However, additional statistical discussion may also be needed in reviewing the decision points and in ensuring that adequate justification exists for selection of a specific dose or narrow dose range. In addition, a justification for the collection of additional biomarker samples, blood, tissue, imaging, etc., in this study to either confirm efficacy or safety results for the existing study, or build knowledge for subsequent research needs, is to be made.

- Formulation specialists are active at this stage providing stability data and preparing sections of the filing which detail the methods for manufacturing the drug. They also contribute to the dose selection discussion.

- Production-plant scientists need to confirm availability of the selected dose and advise the group of any production issues.

- Clinical pharmacologists need to provide an adequate overview of all early clinical issues encountered and contribute to justification of a particular dose or dose range.

- Clinical pharmacokineticists help plan the future population PK studies in phase III and support the biomarker activities.

- Clinical directors (MDs) drive this discussion and make the final decision in selection of the dose or dose range. As before, a decision can be made stating that more information on a particular topic is needed and this information can be obtained concurrent with the ongoing phase III, or if critical before initiation of this study (cochair).

- Marketing representatives update on the market competition and needed product profile.

This once again can be a large meeting with much discussion over all the prior information. As mentioned earlier, there should be no reluctance to go back to early clinical or even preclinical to answer any question raised. There is also significant interaction with the TM scientists as this is the best setting for biomarker research. Balance between this information and conduct of the study should be reached and an agreement made on how and who would be possible blood or tissue donors for such studies (all entered or some subgroup). Plans must also be made to investigate safety and response on special subgroup (e.g., age, gender, or race). As we enter the age of personalized medicine, information on how a drug performs in numerous subgroups will complicate and possibly enlarge these confirmatory studies. The result, however, will improve the understanding of how drugs work when they hit the market.

2.3 TM and Assessment of Biomarkers

The firm contribution that the discipline of TM can make to drug development is the discovery, validation, and interpretation of biomarkers in clinical studies. The promise this makes is that use of these biomarkers will give us earlier evidence for drug activity, either efficacy or safety. Thus, decisions to continue a program, modify the drug, or terminate the program can be made with more certainty than that obtained from results of small studies examining highly varying clinical endpoints. A biomarker is more focused and can give reliable indication of

- Target validation—validating the existence of a disease-related target

- Target/compound interaction—giving us some measure of the level of chemical–physical interaction of the compound drug with the disease-related target

- Pharmacodynamic activity—relating the clinical consequence of the compounds interaction with the disease-related target

- Disease modification—correlating with some degree of change in the status (progression, remission) or presence/absence of the disease

- Disease classification—identifying the different stages of a disease

There are many types of biomarkers (Figure 2.2). Those that are stable and cannot be changed within a patient like genomic, metabolomic, or proteomic biomarkers serve to identify a population and perhaps tailor a specific treatment to that population. They also are useful for discovery efforts. Those that track disease status like imaging and biochemical biomarkers are most useful in tracking changes induced by a treatment, as well as classifying disease status at entry. Yet, some biologic biomarkers are elusive as the basic question of "did the disease give rise to the biomarker or is this biomarker a cause of this disease" always needs to be addressed. To answer this, we need to have a deeper understanding of the disease pathway. For some diseases, this is very difficult to distinguish with certainty. Even for a disease as common as diabetes, we track blood glucose levels or insulin levels as a reliable biomarker for a given treatment. Yet, low insulin and resulting high blood glucose is just a result of the disease. The underlying disease, diabetes, involves the loss or inactivity of insulin-producing cells. Why are there no treatments to change the activity or induce the replacement of these cells? All too often in drug development we focus on treating the symptoms of a disease and not the disease itself.

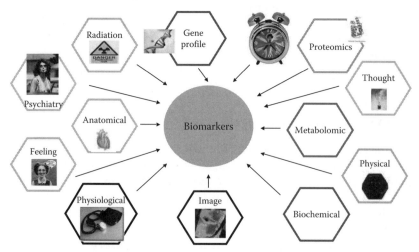

FIGURE 2.2: Biomarkers—plenty to choose from. (From G. Feuerstein, Biomarkers—Plenty to choose from. Original presentation slide, 2007.)

References

Arcy, P.F. and D.W.G. Harron, *Proceedings of The First International Conference on Harmonisation, Brussels 1991*, Queen's University of Belfast, pp. 183–184, 1992.

Chow, S.C. and Liu, J.P. *Statistical Design and Analysis in Pharmaceutical Science: Validation, Process Control, and Stability.* Marcel Dekker, Inc., New York, 1995.

Chow, S.C. and Liu, J.P. *Design and Analysis of Animal Studies in Pharmaceutical Development.* Marcel Dekker, Inc., New York, 1998.

Chow, S.C. and Liu, J.P. *Design and Analysis of Bioavailability and Bioequivalence Studies—Revised and Expanded*, Second edition, Marcel Dekker, Inc., New York, 2000.

Chow, S.C. and Chang, M. *Adaptive Methods in Clinical Trials*, Chapman & Hall/CRC Biostatistics Series. CRC Press, Boca Raton, Florida, 2006.

FDA, *Single Dose Acute Toxicity Testing for Pharmaceuticals; Revised Guidance*, 61 FR 43934 to 43935, August 26, 1996.

FDA draft text, *Guidance for Industry and Reviewers: Estimating the Safe Starting Dose in Clinical Trials for Therapeutics in Adult Healthy Volunteers*, Docket No. 02D–0492, December 2002.

ICH Guidance for Industry (M3). *Nonclinical Safety Studies for the Conduct of Human Clinical Trials for Pharmaceuticals*, July, 1997.

ICH Topic S6 Document, Preclinical Testing of Biotechnology-Derived Pharmaceuticals.

ICH Harmonised Tripartite Guideline (S3A) Note for Toxicokinetics: The Assessment of Systemic Exposure in Toxicity Studies.

ICH Harmonised Tripartite Guideline (S2A) Guidance on Specific Aspects of Regulatory Genotoxicity Tests.

ICH Topic S2B Document, Standard Battery of Genotoxicity Tests.

ICH Harmonised Tripartite Guideline (S1A) Guideline on the Need for Carcinogenicity Studies for Pharmaceuticals.

ICH Harmonised Tripartite Guideline (S5A) Detection of Toxicity to Reproduction for Medicinal Products.

ICH Harmonised Tripartite Guideline (S5B) Toxicity to Male Fertility.

ICH Topic S4 Document, Duration of Chronic Toxicity Testing in Animals (Rodent and Nonrodent Toxicity Testing).

Chapter 3

Design and Analysis Approaches for Discovery Translational Medicine

Dennis Cosmatos and Shein-Chung Chow (Eds.) and Stephen B. Forlow, Jennifer A. Isler, Zhaosheng Lin, and Michael E. Burczynski, with Statistical Appendix by Jessie Q. Xia and S. Stanley Young

Contents

3.1   Introduction

A general understanding of the molecular principles by which diverse types of biomarker assays function can be an important facilitator for optimizing the statistical analyses of biomarker data, generated in translational medicine (TM) studies. The purpose of this chapter is to provide a general overview of various types of biomarker assays, including those analyzing a spectrum of macromolecules ranging from nucleic acids (DNA and RNA) and small-molecule metabolites to larger molecular-weight proteins as analytes.

Biomarker assays can be qualitative, semiquantitative, or quantitative in nature. A common type of qualitative biomarker determination is an assay investigating a single-nucleotide polymorphism (SNP), in which a defined position within a DNA sequence is genotyped on the basis of whether an A, C, G, or T is present at one or more locations within a gene. Qualitative assays employing genotyping methods are described in more detail in Section 3.2.

Semiquantitative determinations come in many different forms and are used in many different applications. Immunohistochemistry (IHC) assays employ a relatively standard 0, 1+, 2+, 3+ scale to indicate the staining intensity of a detection antibody for a specific protein in a slide section. Although newer digital imaging technologies are making IHC assays more quantitative in nature, they are still considered as subjective semiquantitative assays and are often conducted by two independent slide reviewers to strengthen the quality of the measurements. Another example of a semiquantitative assay includes relative RNA-expression measurements using Taqman real-time PCR (in the absence of external or internal standards). In these assays, the difference in the relative levels of an RNA transcript among the samples can be estimated on the basis of a variety of assumptions, provided certain conditions are met. The principles of semiquantitative RNA measurements are also discussed in Section 3.2.

Most high-content biomarker assays (oligonucleotide- or cDNA-based gene arrays, protein arrays, two-dimensional [2D] proteomics gels, etc.) are also considered semiquantitative, as they are designed to screen a large number of analytes and give an approximate "first-pass" indication of the biomarkers that may be useful to measure. After the initial high-content screens geared toward biomarker discovery are conducted using semiquantitative approaches, the results of such biomarker-discovery studies are typically confirmed with the quantitative assays.

All the types of molecular biomarkers covered in this chapter—nucleic acids, proteins, and small-molecule metabolites—can be assessed with either relative or absolute quantitative methods. Transcript measurements can employ either internal or external standards to yield quantitative copy-number results. Enzyme-linked immunosorbent assays (ELISAs) for the determination of peptide or protein levels use the external standards to indicate the concentrations of proteins or peptides in a sample, and LC/MS assays can use internal and/or external standard approaches to quantitatively determine the concentrations of the metabolites in the samples.

The molecular bases and the general types of data output generated by selected assays of each type are presented in the remaining sections of this chapter. It is hoped that this overview, meant not to be comprehensive but rather representative, will familiarize the reader with the molecular foundations for data generation in many biomarker studies, and provide a rationale for implementing the appropriate statistical analyses for the assessment of biomarker data generated by the diverse biomarker-assay technologies.

3.2 Genomic Assays

Genomic assays generally encompass assays designed to detect either DNA or RNA as analytes. DNA-based assays (sometimes also referred to as pharmacogenetic assays) are most often qualitative in nature (i.e., they measure a static genotype), although a semiquantitative aspect can be associated with the qualitative measurement (percent of DNA in a sample appearing to possess a given genotype). Though not specifically addressed in this study, the DNA-based assays can also be quantitative, if the amounts of DNA is measured in an individual subject (for instance, measurements of plasmid vectors as a PK measure employed in a vaccine study, or measurements of shed tumor-DNA in a surrogate tissue, such as serum in advanced cancer patients as a potential measure of the disease status, etc.). As discussed in the introduction, RNA-based assays (also referred to as transcriptional profiling assays) are either semiquantitative or quantitative in nature. The molecular principles by which various targeted genomic assays work are described in the following sections.

3.2.1 Qualitative DNA Genotyping Assays

With the identification of an increasing number of polymorphisms that may predict patient responses and ultimately guide the therapeutic decision-making, there has been a concomitant increase in the number of laboratories (from small clinical sites to dedicated genotyping facilities) that routinely perform genotyping analysis. The basis of all the targeted genotyping assays is PCR amplification of a region containing the polymorphism of interest, although a variety of techniques may be employed, which range from rudimentary processes, such as restriction fragment length polymorphism (RFLP) in which polymorphisms can be detected visually by differences in the restriction-enzyme digestion pattern of genomic DNA upon gel electrophoresis, to advanced technologies such as matrix-assisted laser desorption ionization/time-of-flight mass spectrometry (MALDI-TOF MS), in which detection is based on mass differences of polymorphic and non-polymorphic primer extension products. All the genotyping assays can be applied qualitatively (i.e., identification of the specific nucleotide at the polymorphic position); however, genotyping methods with increased sensitivity are also capable of semiquantitative detection (discussed in the following section). The level of throughput is also an important distinction between genotyping platforms, either at the level of simplex versus multiplex detection (e.g., of single-nucleotide analyses in target genes [PCR-RFLP versus MALDI-TOF MS]) or at an even more comprehensive level, with the ability to perform whole genome-wide scans using DNA array technologies.

3.2.1.1   PCR-RFLP

Perhaps one of the earliest technologies available for polymorphism detection became available shortly after the characterization of restriction enzymes that cleave DNA in a sequence-specific manner. Since even a single nucleotide change in DNA, as is the case with SNPs, can alter a restriction-enzyme recognition site, polymorphisms can be detected by differences in the size of DNA fragments upon digestion with a given restriction enzyme. This is illustrated in the example shown in Figure 3.1a, in which the CYP2C9-*6 allele-defining SNP creates an *Mnl*I restriction site, and thereby alters the pattern of fragments generated upon cleavage with the *Mnl*I enzyme. Figure 3.1b shows an actual agarose-gel image of the *Mnl*I-digested genomic DNA from a subject that does not have the *6 SNP (Subject A) and a subject heterozygous for the *6 SNP (Subject B).

Since PCR-RFLP requires enzymatic digestion of each individual's genomic DNA sequence and subsequent analysis of restriction fragments by agarose-gel electrophoresis, the technique is not only low throughput, but also requires manual inspection by the laboratory technician to compare a given sample's restriction fragment pattern with that of samples with known genotypes, to make a genotype determination. Results are solely qualitative and are often complicated to interpret, because of the differences in the restriction-fragment intensities owing to the incomplete restriction digestion or other gel artifacts that must be subjectively analyzed by the technician for every analytical run.

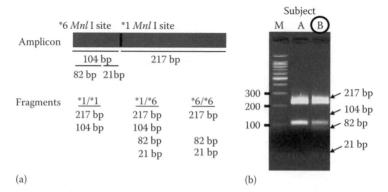

FIGURE 3.1:   PCR-RFLP assays. (a) CYP2C9*6 allele-defining SNP. (b) Agarose gel image of differing alleles of CYP2C9.

3.2.1.2   Primer Extension/MALDI-TOF MS

Primer extension coupled with MALDI-TOF MS-based detection is considered as one of the more advanced, targeted genotyping platforms for several reasons. First, the technology affords high sample-throughput by virtue of its 384-well plate format and the ability to "multiplex" (i.e., simultaneously perform multiple genotyping assays on a single genomic sample). Additionally, complex software associated with the MALDI-TOF instrumentation assigns genotype calls with little to no intervention by the technician. Briefly, analysis of polymorphisms using primer extension assays coupled with MALDI-TOF MS analysis entails three major steps: (1) PCR amplification of the sequence containing the polymorphic site, (2) primer extension through the polymorphic site in the presence of a combination of deoxynucleotide triphosphates (dNTPs) and ddNTPs, and (3) MALDI-TOF analysis of the primer-extended products. This principle is presented graphically in Figure 3.2a and details of the protocol are described below.

After amplifying a region of the genomic DNA containing the polymorphic site of interest, shrimp alkaline phosphatase is added to dephosphorylate the residual nucleotides from the PCR reaction prior to initiating the primer extension reaction. In the next step, an extension reaction employs a primer that anneals to the PCR amplicon and is located with its 3′ end juxtaposed to the polymorphic site. Addition of a "termination mix" (containing a specified combination of nonterminating dNTPs and chain-terminating ddNTPs) to initiate the primer extension reaction causes dNTPs to be incorporated until a sequence-dependent ddNTP incorporation event terminates the reaction. Since the termination point and number of nucleotides incorporated are sequence-specific, the mass of the extension products can be used to identify the nucleotide present at the polymorphic site. Primer mass-spectra data is directly converted into genotype calls using a software that assigns confidence levels for each call, based on the peak characteristics, including the closeness of the observed atomic masses with the expected masses of primer extension products in the sample and the signal-to-noise ratios observed for each of the peaks. An example of the raw spectra generated from a multiplexed MALDI-TOF assay in which three polymorphic positions were interrogated in a single assay is shown in Figure 3.2b. In this example, the sample was determined to be wild-type with respect to all the three alleles tested, as shown by only a single peak (indicated by colored arrows) at the location of each wild-type extended primer.

3.2.1.3   Taqman Allelic Discrimination

Taqman allelic discrimination assays utilize real-time PCR technology, similar to that used for quantitative gene-expression analysis. Allelic discrimination technology is moderate in terms of sample throughput, since, like MALDI-TOF MS, it can be performed in 384-well format; however, it is not amenable to multiplexing. The assay utilizes a standard pair of PCR primers to amplify a region containing the polymorphism of interest and two detection probes that are differentially labeled with fluorescent dyes and bind to either the non-polymorphic or the polymorphic sequence. The schematic shown in Figure 3.3a illustrates the principle of allelic

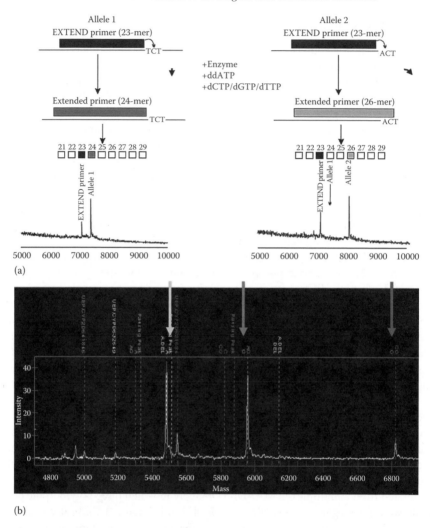

FIGURE 3.2: (See color insert following page 146.) Analysis of polymorphisms using primer extension assays coupled with MALDI-TOF MS analysis.

discrimination. When bound to its complimentary sequence, the probe is cleaved by DNA polymerase during PCR amplification and its fluorescence signal is emitted. Unbound probes do not fluoresce, and therefore, the genotype of the target sequence is determined based on the fluorescence profile of each sample.

Allelic discrimination software plots the fluorescence values for each detection probe in each sample using a cluster plot, in which the 2D location of each sample is determined by the strength of fluorescence for each of the detection probes. An algorithm assigns a confidence score for each genotype call, based on the "closeness" of each sample with other samples exhibiting similar fluorescence properties.

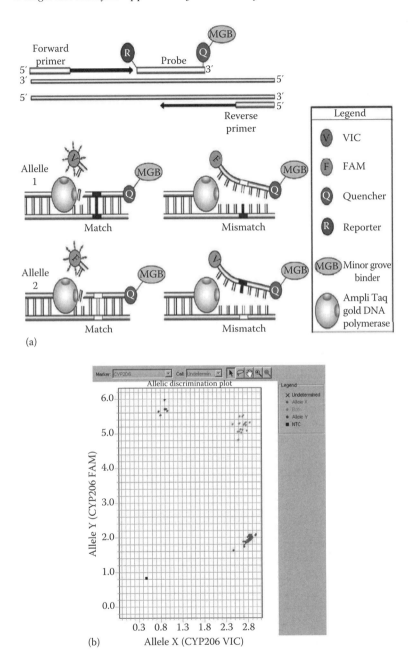

FIGURE 3.3: (See color insert following page 146.) Taqman allelic discrimination. (a) Allelic discrimination using PCR amplification with two PCR primers. (b) Cluster plot showing fluorescence patterns for homozygote samples for Allele X (red) and Allele Y (blue), and XY heterozygotes (green).

Homozygotes for one allele show increased fluorescence in one channel and baseline fluorescence in the other, while heterozygotes possessing both the alleles exhibit intermediate fluorescence in both channels. Figure 3.3b shows an example of a cluster plot in which homozygote samples for Allele X and Allele Y are shown in red and blue, respectively, and heterozygote samples are shown in green.

3.2.1.4   Pyrosequencing

Pyrosequencing differs from many other methods, as it provides genotyping results in the context of the neighboring DNA sequence. The technology affords moderate sample-throughput as the samples are run in 96-well format and multiplexing is rare, although it can be accomplished at very low levels upon careful optimization. Following PCR amplification of the target DNA sequence, a sequencing primer is hybridized to a biotinylated single-stranded template using streptavidin beads. In a series of enzymatic events (illustrated in Figure 3.4a) dNTPs are incorporated into the extending primer and each incorporation event is accompanied by the release of pyrophosphate, which ultimately generates visible light in amounts proportional to the amount of incorporated nucleotide. The light emitted is detected by a camera and visualized as a peak in a pyrogram.

Pyrosequencing software calculates peak heights upon addition of each nucleotide, and genotypes are determined by comparison with the predicted theoretical pyrograms. Genotype calls are assigned quality scores of pass, check, or fail, based on a number of factors, including the agreement between the theoretical and actual pyrograms, observed signal-to-noise ratios, and calculated peak widths. As the light emission is proportional to the amount of nucleotide incorporated, the pyrosequencing platform can provide semiquantitative determination, such as the percentage of a given polymorphism in a mixed population or the number of gene copies in a genomic sample. An example of a theoretical pyrogram and the actual pyrogram for a sample bearing the predicted genotype are presented in Figure 3.4b.

3.2.2   Semiquantitative DNA Mutation Assays

As previously mentioned, technological platforms, such as MALDI-TOF MS and pyrosequencing, offer the advantage of quantifying DNA, based on single-nucleotide differences. This type of quantitative detection is a unique and powerful tool that allows one to assess the percentage of a specific DNA sequence within a heterogeneous sample population. Semiquantitative mutation assays have multiple applications that include monitoring the evolution of mutant viral strains within a subject, assessing the frequency of an allele or mutation within a single pooled-DNA sample representing many different subjects, and quantitatively measuring the amount of mutant DNA within a heterogeneous tumor sample. Quantitative measurements using a genotyping platform rely on the fact that the signal generated, for example, mass peak-height for MALDI-TOF MS or the light intensity for pyrosequencing, is proportional to the amount of variant DNA sequence detected in the sample.

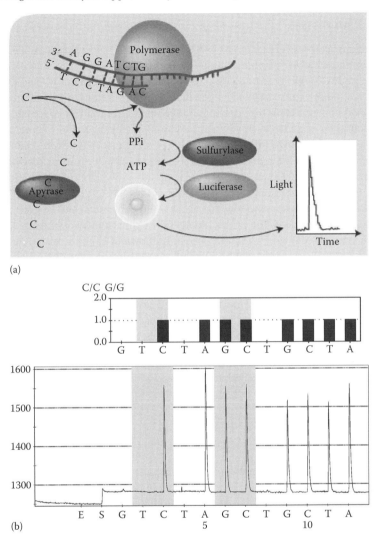

(a)

(b)

FIGURE 3.4:   Pyrosequencing assays. (a) Enzymatic events lead to emission of pyrophosphate and visible light; (b) Theoretical (top) and actual (bottom) pyrogram.

Therefore, by comparing the signals of wild-type sequence with the mutant one, a relative percentage can be calculated. The sensitivity of the technique is a critical factor in quantitation, and the limit of detection (LOD) for most quantitative genotyping assays is typically around 10%–15%, a significant improvement over the convention DNA-sequencing approaches ($\sim$25%).

3.2.3   RNA Assays

By measuring the level of RNA transcripts in a cell (or multiple types of cells), one can determine whether specific genes are up- or downregulated, for example, during disease progression or in response to a therapeutic drug. In effect, by characterizing the levels of gene expression under specific conditions, a transcriptional profile can be obtained that can form the basis of a "signature." Microarray approaches allow many thousands of genes to be interrogated simultaneously, and are therefore considered as the most powerful tools available for screening gene-expression profiles of biological samples. However, these initial screens must be followed up with techniques that confirm and quantitatively measure the expression of candidate genes, most commonly by quantitative real-time PCR (qRT-PCR).

qRT-PCR assays use gene-specific amplification primers and a gene-specific fluorescence-labeled detection probe to detect the expression level of its target gene. The detection probe is labeled with a $5'$-FAM reporter dye and a $3'$-nonfluorescent quencher. As PCR product is amplified, the $5'$-nuclease activity of DNA polymerase releases the reporter dye from its proximity to the quencher, allowing fluorescence. This fluorescence is captured in real time and plotted on an amplification plot. When the amplification plot crosses the threshold (a level above the baseline, but low enough to be within the exponential growth region of the amplification plot), a cycle threshold (Ct) is determined. Implicit in the qRT-PCR approach is the ability to accurately measure the RNA levels, either semiquantitatively or quantitatively, using standards and normalization strategies, several of which are described in the following sections.

3.2.4   Semiquantitative RNA Assays

3.2.4.1   Delta-Ct Approach

By definition, a delta-Ct approach relies on the difference in the Ct values between two genes in the same sample or between a gene in two samples. For example, "control" genes, whose expression has been determined to be relatively stable under the desired conditions, are often used to normalize the measurements of other genes to more accurately compare the gene expression among different samples. By subtracting the Ct value of a control gene (or the mean of several control genes), a delta-Ct can be calculated for all target genes. These values can then be used to evaluate gene-expression changes between the samples by subtracting the delta-Ct in one sample from the delta-Ct in the other (i.e., the delta–delta-Ct). Since PCR amplification is exponential, the fold difference between the normalized levels of the target gene in different samples is approximated by the following formula:

$$\text{Fold difference} = 2^{\wedge}(\Delta \text{Ctsample1} - \Delta \text{Ctsample2})$$

One caveat to this approach is that it relies on 100% efficiency for PCR amplification, which is rarely the case. Moreover, the methods are incapable of giving any information about the actual copy numbers of the target transcripts measured.

3.2.5 Taqman Low-Density Arrays

Taqman low-density arrays (TLDAs) represent one of the most high-throughput methods for semiquantitative measurement of RNA transcripts. The TLDA is a 384-well microfluidics card enabling 384 real-time PCR reactions to be performed simultaneously. Each TLDAs contains eight ports or reservoirs, each having 48 connected wells preloaded with Taqman gene-expression assays, allowing between one and eight samples to be analyzed depending on the number of different assays contained on each card. The assays for multiple control genes are included to allow gene expression to be normalized within a sample to facilitate the comparison of gene expression measurements across the samples.

3.2.6 Quantitative RNA Assays

External and internal standard approaches represent the most quantitative approaches available in qRT-PCR today, and enable users to calculate copy numbers of the target transcripts, if the appropriate standards are used.

3.2.7 External Standard-Based Quantitative RNA Assays

DNA-based external standard curves involve the quantification of a plasmid bearing the DNA of interest and the extrapolation of an unknown sample's C_T value to this standard curve to determine the copy number. In this approach, a known quantity of DNA corresponding to the RNA sequence of interest is quantified by UV spectrophotometry, such that the copy number (in terms of double-stranded DNA) can be calculated. Unknown samples are reverse-transcribed, and then PCR amplified alongside the plasmid DNA standard curve. Since the plasmid DNA standard curve is PCR amplified with the samples, the PCR efficiency can be calculated, with the assumption that PCR amplification efficiency is similar for both the standards and the samples. However, any discrepancies in the efficiencies for the reverse-transcription reactions that generate samples and standards can have a significant impact on the plasmid DNA-based quantitation, since following exponential amplification, the effects on quantitation can be quite large.

RNA-based external standard curves represent a more rigorous external standard approach for accurate RNA quantitation, although even this method has its limitations. This method involves the reverse transcription and PCR amplification of unknown samples, alongside a standard curve composed of known quantities of the RNA of interest. Extrapolation of the unknown sample's C_T value from this standard curve can be used to determine the copy number in terms of the starting RNA molecules. In this approach, the RNA standard is generated by *in vitro* transcription from a purified DNA template, and quantified by UV spectrophotometry such that the copy number (in terms of single-stranded RNA) can be calculated. Both unknown samples and standards are reverse-transcribed and PCR amplified in the same assay. Since the RNA standard curve is both reverse-transcribed and PCR-amplified with the samples, the overall RT-PCR efficiency can be calculated. The only assumption that this method makes is the assumption that is inherent to all external standard-based approaches, namely, that the overall RT-PCR efficiency is the same for both the samples and standards in the individual wells within an assay or analytical run.

3.2.8   Internal Standard-Based Quantitative RNA Assays

Internal standard-based approaches using DNA internal standards are subjected to the same caveats regarding potential variation in the RT efficiency between the samples, since the internal standardization only occurs during PCR. Nonetheless, these methods are extremely quantitative in terms of characterizing the efficiency of PCR amplification. Internal standard methods are the only approaches that do not require the assumption that the overall PCR efficiency is the same between the samples and the external standards. Rather, the efficiency of amplification in each sample is well documented by virtue of the measurable extent of the internal standard amplification. Thus, internal standard approaches can adjust for the variable presence of PCR inhibitors or other phenomena that may confound qRT-PCR analyses.

Genomic assays can be designed to

1. Query nucleotide sequences within the critical genes to determine whether they will be functional or nonfunctional (qualitative DNA genotyping assays)

2. Determine relative amounts of mutated sequences amongst nonmutated sequences (semiquantitative DNA assays)

3. Compare relative levels of RNA transcripts between two or more samples (semiquantitative RNA assays)

4. Quantitate the absolute copy numbers of the RNA transcripts in the individual samples (quantitative RNA assays)

A number of detection methodologies can be employed to measure these types of biomarkers and only a small number are reviewed in this study. Innovation in the field of nucleic acid analysis continues to increase, and the adoption and use of DNA and RNA biomarkers as pharmacogenetic and pharmacogenomic biomarkers in the translational studies will certainly expand in the coming years.

3.3   Immunoassays

Immunoassays are used extensively within the TM and clinical studies for biomarker measurements. Immunoassays are designed to specifically detect and quantify the concentrations of analytes (i.e., proteins, peptides, hormones, and antibodies) in a biological sample. Valuable biomarker data can be obtained by applying immunoassays in various biological matrices, including serum, plasma, synovial fluid, sputum, cerebrospinal fluid, bronchoalveolar lavage, and urine.

The basis of all immunoassays is the ability to adsorb an antibody or an analyte to a solid surface (e.g., wells of a polystyrene microtiter plate or $\sim$5 μM polystyrene microspheres/beads) and still retain its specific high-affinity binding function. Immunoassays are typically performed in standard 96- or 384-well polystyrene microtiter plates. Traditionally, immunoassays that utilize coated wells of a microtiter plate can detect one analyte per sample. However, the advanced immunoassay technology uses plate-based immunoassay arrays or multiplexed assays. Plate-based multiplexed assays are created by spotting up to 25 different capture antibodies per well in a 96-well plate, which enables the detection and quantitation of up to 25 analytes per sample. Recently, another emerging technology is the bead-based immunoassay platforms, which have become heavily utilized owing to their solution-phase kinetics and their ability to multiplex. Various companies have produced bead-based assays that can measure anywhere from a single analyte up to 100 analytes per sample.

Regardless of the immunoassay platform, the most common immunoassay format to specifically detect and quantify an analyte is the sandwich assay (Figure 3.5).

Sandwich immunoassays require capture and detection antibodies that recognize two nonoverlapping epitopes on the analyte. The antibodies are the major factor determining the sensitivity and specificity of an immunoassay. The antibodies specific for the analyte can be either monoclonal or polyclonal, but monoclonal antibodies generally improve the specificity of the assay.

In a sandwich assay, the capture antibody is coated onto the surface of the wells of a microtiter plate or a bead. Following sample addition, the analyte in the sample is bound by the capture antibody. After washing, a detection antibody is added to form a "sandwich," which enables the quantification of analyte using various detection methods (see below). For multiplexed bead-based assays, the specific analyte is distinguished by the bead fluorophore and the level of the analyte is quantified, based on the amount of detection antibody, like a typical sandwich immunoassay.

Competitive immunoassays constitute another type of immunoassay format. Competitive immunoassays are typically employed in certain situations, such as when two

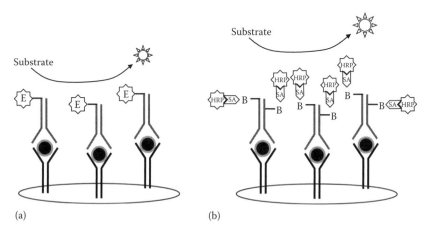

FIGURE 3.5: Sandwich immunoassays. (a) Direct sandwich ELISA, and (b) indirect sandwich ELISA.

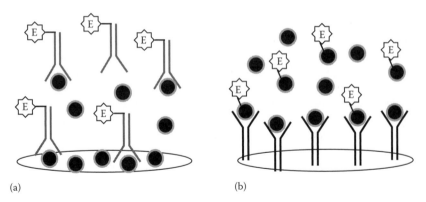

(a)   (b)

FIGURE 3.6:   Competitive immunoassays. (a) Labeled antibody, and (b) labeled analyte.

antibodies recognizing nonoverlapping epitopes have not been identified, or when the analyte is small and might only possess a single antibody-binding site. Competitive assays can be implemented using two different approaches (Figure 3.6). One approach is to coat the surface of a plate with the analyte of interest. The detection antibody is added along with the sample onto the plate, and the unlabeled analyte in the sample competes with the plate-bound analyte for binding to the detection antibody. Higher analyte concentrations in the sample result in lower response signals, owing to lower detection antibody binding to the coated analyte (Figure 3.6a). Another approach is to coat the wells of the plate with capture antibody. The analyte is labeled and added with the sample. Unlabeled analyte in the sample competes with the labeled analyte for binding to the capture antibody on the plate. Higher analyte concentrations in the sample result in lower response signals generated from the bound labeled analyte (Figure 3.6b).

Immunoassays can also be designed to quantify active analyte in a sample. A capture activity immunoassay can be designed by coating an antibody to the analyte of interest on the wells of a microtiter plate, to bind the analyte in the sample (Figure 3.7a). An important requirement for this type of assay is the use of a capture antibody that does not inhibit the activity of the captured analyte. This type of assay is set up such that the antibody-bound analyte can modify the activity of a labeled detection reagent or substrate (e.g., upregulating or downregulating enzyme activity upon binding) added by the user. Upon activation by the analyte, the added substrate becomes detectable and correlates to the level of analyte captured by the original capture antibody (Figure 3.7b).

Although immunoassay platforms and formats have been standard for sometime, new detection method technology has improved the immunoassay sensitivity, dynamic range of measurement, and both the sample and antibody conservation. The most common detection method for immunoassays utilizes an enzymatic reaction. These immunoassays are termed ELISAs. After the capture antibody in this system binds the analyte of interest, a detection enzyme is used that may be either directly conjugated to the detection antibody (Figure 3.5a) or to a secondary antibody that recognizes the detection antibody. However, most often the enzyme is introduced

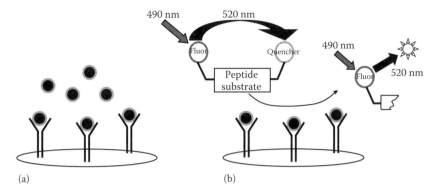

FIGURE 3.7: Capture activity immunoassays. (a) Capture of analyte, and (b) modification of added substrate by active analyte.

indirectly through an avidin–biotin complex to amplify the signal and enhance the detection. For example, a detection antibody can be biotinylated at multiple sites and can bind multiple streptavidin molecules, each of which is labeled with the enzymatic molecule (e.g., HRP (Figure 3.5b)). Detection and quantification is accomplished by incubating the enzyme-complex with a substrate that produces a detectable product.

The choice of substrate for ELISA assays is determined by the required sensitivity level of detection. Enzyme-labeled reagents can be detected using chromogenic, chemifluorescent, and chemiluminescent substrates. Chromogenic substrates generate a soluble, color product that results in a change in the optical density detectable by a spectrophotometer. These colorimetric assays generally provide suitable sensitivity (picogram per milliliter) and dynamic range. Chemiluminescent signals emit light that is measured by a luminometer, whereas fluorescent substrates require excitation for light to be emitted and detected by a fluorometer. Chemifluorescent and chemiluminescent substrates typically yield better sensitivity (<1 pg/mL), a larger linear range of detection, and antibody conservation.

Alternative detection methods include direct fluorescence, electrochemiluminescence (ECL), and fluorescence resonance energy transfer (FRET). As the name implies, with direct fluorescence, the detection antibody is directly labeled with a fluorochrome. ECL is a detection method in which reactive species are generated from stable precursors at the surface of an electrode. ECL is a form of chemiluminescence in which the light-emitting chemiluminescent reaction is preceded by an electrochemical reaction. ECL is highly sensitive (femtomole per liter), shows a wide dynamic range (over 6 orders of magnitude), and utilizes labels that are extremely stable. The FRET detection technique can be applied to capture activity assays to quantify the active analyte in a sample using a fluorescent readout (Figure 3.7). A substrate linked to a fluorochrome and a quencher produces no signal until the substrate is cleaved or the conformation is altered by active analyte. The resulting fluorescent signal can be obtained over time (kinetic readout) or at a defined time after the enzymatic reaction is initiated (end point).

Regardless of the immunoassay assay platform, format, or detection method, the quantification of the analyte in a biological sample is determined using calibrators of known concentrations. The calibrators are generally prepared by spiking recombinant analyte into a calibrator diluent that mimics the biological matrix. The concentration–response relationship is generated by plotting the final response value (OD, median fluorescence, light intensity) against the calibrator concentration (Figure 3.8). The best regression model is determined for fitting a curve to the calibrator concentration–response data. For many immunoassays, a four- or a five-parameter logistic fit are the most appropriate regression models to generate a calibration curve. A typical calibration curve for a sandwich ELISA is shown in Figure 3.8. From the fitted curve, the analyte concentration (e.g., picogram per milliliter, nanomole per liter) in the unknown samples is determined by reading the unknown sample response signal from the calibration curve (Figure 3.8). The intensity of the response signal produced (optical density, fluorescence, light intensity) in a sandwich immunoassay correlates to the concentration of the detection antibody and therefore the analyte concentration. For competitive assays, the response signal produced is inversely proportional to the analyte concentration.

Immunoassays enable highly specific quantitative biomarker data to be acquired from a wide range of biological matrices. Emerging technology platforms and improved detection systems have greatly enhanced the sensitivity of immunoassays, increasing the number of analytes that can be accurately quantitated in human clinical samples. The number of commercially available immunoassays continues to expand and these assays are very amenable to the in-house development. In addition, the introduction of multiplexed assays and the application of automation have increased the throughput of these types of clinical biomarker assays. On the basis of these continuing innovations, it is certain that immunoassays will continue to be a heavily utilized biomarker platform in support of human clinical studies.

3.4   Small-Molecule Metabolite Assays

Small-molecule metabolites generally refer to either metabolites of drugs or endogenous molecules, such as metabolites of proteins, lipids, or hormones. The most commonly used technologies for the analysis of these molecules, includes high-performance liquid chromatography (HPLC), liquid chromatography/mass spectrometry (LC-MS), and liquid chromatography and tandem mass spectrometry (LC-MS/MS). Among these platforms, LC-MS/MS has become increasingly popular not only because of its highly specific nature for both qualitative and quantitative assays, but also owing to its minimal requirement of chromatographic separation of analytes in highly complex samples. In addition to LC-separation-based methods, there are also other less-commonly used technologies for quantitative assays of small-molecule metabolites, such as Surface-enhanced laser desorption ionization/time-of-flight mass spectrometry (SELDI-TOF MS). One advantage of using SELDI technology is its suitability for analyzing small peptides that may be too large and difficult to analyze using a LC-MS/MS approach. The following sections describe the fundamental principles of the manner in which LC-MS/MS and SELDI-TOF are used to perform quantitative or semiquantitative biomarker assays.

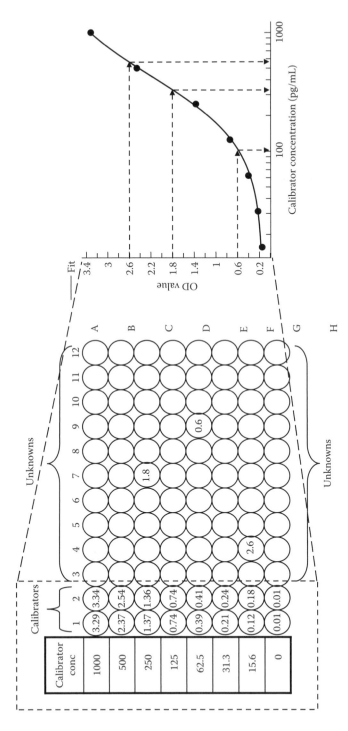

FIGURE 3.8:   A calibrator spiked with recombinant analyte (left) generates response values plotted against known concentrations and a curve is fit to the data (right).

3.4.1 Quantitative LC-MS/MS Assays

With the integration and improvement of different ionization technologies, small molecules with various chemical properties (including polar, nonpolar, basic, acidic, or neutral molecules) can now be analyzed by LC-MS/MS. LC-MS/MS assays utilize both HPLC or LC and tandem mass spectrometry (MS/MS) technologies to analyze small-molecule metabolites in complex biological samples. As the biological samples may contain thousands or more of different compounds with a wide range of molecular properties, achieving sufficient separation of the target analyte from other entities in the sample matrix is critical to the specificity and sensitivity of LC-MS/MS assays. HPLC can separate the target analytes from many (but not all) other compounds, based on its retention time on a chosen column, which can greatly reduce the matrix effect and allow the measurement of multiple analytes in a single assay by the mass spectrometer.

Sometimes, an initial purification step, such as solid phase extraction (SPE) can be employed, which can simultaneously purify and enrich an analyte extracted from an original sample. The dual goals of using SPE prior to LC-MS/MS are to (1) quickly clean up or purify the samples and (2) concentrate target analytes in the sample in a suitable volume for the following LC-MS/MS analysis. The principle of SPE is similar to that of HPLC, which includes binding of certain types of compounds in the sample to the chosen solid phase in a column and elution of these compounds from the solid phase using selective buffers. After the analyte has been separated from many of the components in the sample mixture by SPE and/or LC, MS/MS is employed to further isolate the analyte of interest and allow its quantitation.

The first step of MS/MS analysis is proper ionization of the target analytes. Depending on the molecular properties of the analytes (polar or nonpolar, basic, acidic, or neutral), different ionization methods, including ESI (electrospray ionization), APPI (atmospheric pressure photo ionization), and APCI (atmospheric chemical ionization) can be utilized. Both positive and negative ions may be generated during the ionization process: addition of proton(s) to an analyte produces positive ion(s) and loss of proton(s) from an analyte generates negative ion(s). Only an ionized analyte can be detected and quantified by a mass spectrometer.

The quantitation of an ionized analyte is normally performed in a typical triple quadrupole MS system. The triple quadrupole MS system consists of three quadrupoles in tandem, named Q1, Q2, and Q3. The Q1 quadrupole functions as a selective filter to allow the entry of selected precursor ion(s) with specified mass/charge (m/z) ratios. The Q2 quadrupole acts as a collision cell providing an environment for the filtered precursor ion(s) to collide with an inert gas and to generate fragments or product ions of the precursor ion(s). The fragmentation process in Q2 is generally termed CID (collision-induced dissociation). In the final quadrupole (Q3), product ion(s) of interest are monitored or selected. The ionization process of analytes and their analysis by a triple quadrupole tandem mass spectrometer is depicted in Figure 3.9. In quadrupole LC-MS assays, analytes in the sample are quantitated, based on the measured ion transitions between the initially filtered precursor ion of interest captured in Q1, and the fragment ion (daughter ion) that is produced after CID in Q2.

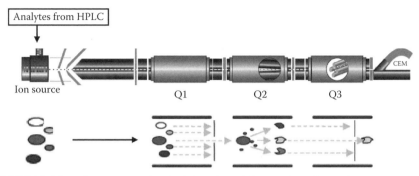

FIGURE 3.9: Structure and principle of a triple quadrupole tandem mass spectrometer. Separated analytes from HPLC are ionized and sprayed into the mass spectrometer as very fine charged droplets (shown as colored spheres) by high voltage and heated gas. One or more target precursor ions may be selected in Q1 based on their molecular masses (*m/z* ratio). Fragmentation of selected precursor ion(s) occur in Q2 by a mechanism called CID. Selected product ion(s) (fragment or daughter ion) may be monitored by Q3.

The most frequently used MS/MS mode for quantitative assay is multiple reaction monitoring (MRM), which measures the transition of a precursor ion to one or more of its characteristic fragment ions. This approach ensures the most specific and sensitive measurement of analytes by LC-MS applications. In most cases, an internal standard is applied to the sample during the initial sample processing step, which allows the measured analyte concentration to be back-calculated based on the recovery of the internal standard. The most suitable internal standards are deuterated or ^{13}C labeled analytes, because they share identical or similar chemical properties of the analytes and yet can be differentiated from the analytes in MS spectra by their molecular masses.

One such example is the quantitative assay for isoprostanes by LC-MS/MS. Isoprostanes are prostaglandin isomers that are commonly used as oxidative-stress biomarkers in different biological matrices. The molecular weight of isoprostanes is 354, with a singly charged negative ion (de-protonated precursor ion) at m/z (mass/ charge ratio) of 353 (Figure 3.10a). The MS/MS fragment spectrum of the isoprostane precursor ion shows a characteristic fragment ion at m/z of 193.1 (Figure 3.10b). A deuterated isoprostane with 4 or more protons replaced by deuterium (MW + 4) can be used as the internal standard. Thus, ion transition from 353 to 193.1 (353/193.1) can be measured to acquire quantitative data for the isoprostane. Multiple ion transitions can be monitored and measured within the same assay as demonstrated in Figure 3.10c, and depicted as a total ion chromatogram (TIC), showing retention times and ion intensities of multiple ion transitions over time (353/193.1 for 8-isoprostanes or iPF2α-III, and 353/115.0 for both iPF2α-VI and 8,12-iso-iPF2α-VI) within the same LC-MS/MS assay. The ratio between the peak areas of these transitions relative to the internal standard's ion transition provides the information needed to quantitate each isoprostane isomer in a sample, after comparison with the peak area ratios between the known calibrator standards and the internal standard.

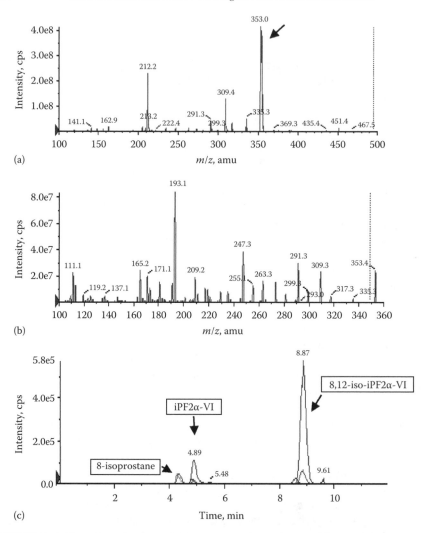

FIGURE 3.10: Quantitation of isoprostanes by LC-MS/MS: (a) full MS scan showing a precursor ion of 8-isoprostane; (b) full MS/MS scan showing fragment ions of 8-isoprostane; and (c) LC-MS/MS chromatogram showing retention of isoprostanes.

3.4.2 SELDI-TOF Assay for Small Peptides

SELDI-TOF is another useful tool to determine the molecular weights and relative abundance of metabolites below or around 10 kd. When combined with an antibody-enriched step, SELDI-TOF assays for one or more analytes can be semiquantitative or quantitative (with the application of internal standards). The key step of SELDI is the application of various chip surfaces (Figure 3.11a) that are capable of selectively

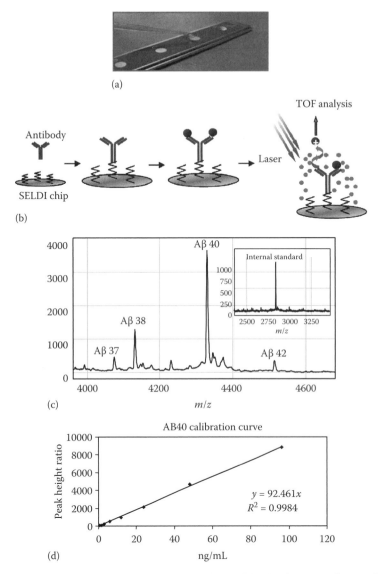

FIGURE 3.11: Quantitation of beta-amyloid peptides by SELDI-TOF: (a) SELDI chip; (b) antibody-captured SELDI-TOF process; (c) Aβ peptides in human CSF detected by SELDI-TOF; and (d) a calibration curve for quantitation of Aβ 40 by SELDI-TOF.

capturing proteins or peptides for analysis. For example, antibodies may be utilized on a chip surface that allows enrichment of target peptides from complex samples. Figure 3.11b shows the procedure of an antibody based capture SELDI-TOF assay. The analyte-specific antibody is first linked to the chip through covalent binding. Sample is then added onto the chip to allow binding of target analytes by the captured antibody. Addition of matrix and the application of laser subsequently causes the flight or desorption (release) of the ionized analyte. The molecular mass of the analyte is calculated based on the flight speed of the ionized analyte within the TOF mass analyzer.

One such example of this type of assay is the quantitation of β-amyloid peptides that are analyzed as biomarkers in Alzheimer's disease. A monoclonal antibody recognizing the common N-terminus of these peptides is used to capture and enrich the β-amyloid peptides from the biological samples on the SELDI-TOF chip surface. Figure 3.11c is a SELDI-TOF spectrum showing simultaneous detection of multiple beta-amyloid peptides sharing homologous N-terminal sequence. Specificity of the assay is ensured through both antibody recognition and the measured molecular masses of detected peaks matching the known molecular weights of β-amyloid peptides. Semiquantitative data are obtained by comparing the relative abundance of peptide ions (reflected by peak heights) between samples, while quantitative data (e.g., nanogram per milliliter) can be determined by calculating the peak height ratio of β-amyloid peptide versus an internal standard (as described previously) and comparing the ratio in a sample with those of known calibrators used in a calibration curve (Figure 3.11d). One disadvantage of using SELDI-TOF versus LC-MS/MS for quantitative assays is that this platform appears less stable and exhibits less reproducible performance over time, which may be owing to the chip surface stability, mass spectrometer instrument, or both. The consequences are generally lower precision and accuracy (higher %CV and Bias) that are very important parameters of assay performance.

3.5   Conclusions

Appropriate statistical analysis in all of the above-mentioned scenarios (and others) is vital to utilize immunoassay biomarker data to properly understand and interpret the data, and to make informative clinical drug-development decisions at critical junctures of clinical programs. It is hoped that by providing an understanding of the molecular aspects by which these biomarker assays work, the development of effective statistical analysis plans for biomarker data generated by these platforms will be greatly facilitated. Some statistical approaches for analyses of these types of data are suggested in the Appendix section.

Statistical Appendix*

A.3.1   Analysis of Gene-Expression Data

As mentioned, gene expression using high-throughput methodologies is a central technology for discovery in biology. Techniques, such as microarray hybridization,

---

* The appendix was contributed by Jessie Q. Xia and S. Stanley Young.

allow the simultaneous quantification of tens of thousands of gene transcripts. The Gene Expression Omnibus, GEO, from the National Center for Biotechnology Information, NCBI, is a public repository that archives over 7000 experiments, over 120,000 data arrays, and over three billion individual data items addressing a wide range of biological questions (Wheeler et al. 2007). The GEO high-throughput gene expression-data submitted by the scientific community is freely available with a web download. The GEO is accessible at www.ncbi.nlm.gov/geo. The GEO data may be freely explored, queried, and visualized to address specific biological or toxicological questions. It makes economic sense to use the existing data rather than rerun an experiment. There may be reasons for rerunning an experiment: new and better gene chips could become available or one might not want to depend on the experimental execution or analysis of the original investigators. Even if the same or similar experiment is carried out, it makes sense to use GEO data to help design the new experiment and to confirm claims from the new experiment.

Perhaps just as important, and possibly unappreciated, the GEO data sets can serve as a self-teaching material for learning statistical and visualization methods used to understand these complex data sets. Most of the data sets in GEO point to a literature paper that can serve as a guide to those wanting to learn how to analyze the corresponding complex data. The main purpose of this work is to reanalyze a GEO data set and to go through the thinking process that goes into such an analysis. We attempt to present this work at an entry level for biologists wanting to learn more about analysis and visualization, and for informatics specialists wanting to have a clear analysis strategy.

For our analysis, we used the Array Studio v2.0. A demo version is freely available from www.omicsoft.com. This software has a rather complete set of analysis and visualization tools. It also has a "one-click" download of GEO data sets. For an experiment, there are actually at least three data sets of interest (see Figure A.3.1).

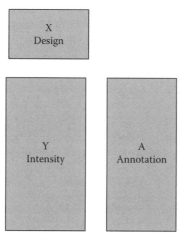

FIGURE A.3.1:   Data sets of interest generated by a typical microarray experiment.

Of course, there is the assay data of interest as well. This is usually formatted as a table where each row is a gene and each column is a sample. The analysis software has to know how the samples are related with one another. These relationships and any other descriptions of the samples are in a "design" data set. Each column of the design is linked to a corresponding column in the assay data set. It is essentially impossible to know the story behind each gene (probe set); hence, the third data set is the annotation data set that is available from the microarray platform provider. Each row of the annotation data set corresponds to a gene, and pertinent information on that gene is stored in the row of A. The three data sets, X (design), Y (assay intensities), and A (annotations) are linked forming what we call a "L" data set. Our presentation does not assume the use of Array Studio, but for convenience, we used it as the demo version can be freely downloaded.

There are many ways to learn. Often in school, we read about what we are to learn. We study the theory. We wait for a long time to actually practice what we are learning. If a young child wants to be a doctor, he/she will be in mid-twenties before he/she does much doctoring and in his/her thirties, before having the real doctoring responsibilities. New theories of language learning emphasize practical approach versus book study, and getting everything correct before you speak the new language. In this study we took a data set (and a corresponding paper from the published literature) from the GEO. The paper which we obtained was concerned with iron uptake in CaCo-2 cells and is fully described in the following section. By reanalysis of this data set, we try to emphasize that learning by practical approach is a good way to become skilled in the analysis of microarray data. One should not wait until everything is understood to start the analysis of a data set.

A.3.2   Analysis of a Sample Data Set

Chicault et al. (2006) (hereafter CTM), studied the effect of iron, in excess and deficit on gene expression in CaCo-2 cells. Regulation of iron absorption by intestinal cells is essential for the maintenance of homeostasis of iron by preventing iron deficiency or overload. The CaCo-2 cells are derived from the intestine, and hence, act as the natural model for the study of iron absorption, and more details are given with this regard can be obtained from their paper. We summarize their experiment to motivate the statistical analysis that we present. The intention of CTM was to mimic iron overload, a normal iron level, and an iron deficit. Their experimental conditions are displayed in a 2×2 data table (Table A.3.1). This figure has the appearance of a 2×2 factorial experiment, the factors being base medium, DMEM or IMDM, and iron, not added or supplemental (hemin or ferric ammonium citrate,

TABLE A.3.1:   Model 2×2 factorial table—model or abstract.

	Factor 2	
Factor 1	**Level 1**	**Level 2**
Level 1	1	2
Level 2	3	4

TABLE A.3.2:   Four treatments are used to ascertain the effects of iron on CaCo-2 cell gene expression. Two media types are used. Three iron physiologic states are mimicked.

Group	Base Media	Serum Supp.	Iron Supp.	Physiological State	Nonheme Iron (μM)	Intracellular Ferritin
1	DMEN	FBS	0	Normal	3.5	11.9
2	DMEN	FBS	Hemin	Iron overload	3.1	1074.0
3	IMDM	Syn mix	0	Iron deficient	0.1	9.4
4	IMDM	Syn mix	FAC	Normal	3.0	85.9

FAC). Their experimental details give a much more complex reality. One might mistakenly think that groups 1 and 3 are iron deficient, based on the margin labels. In fact, group 1 is at a normal iron level as fetal bovine serum (FBS) contains iron, whereas group 3 is iron deficient, as the synthetic growth factors that replace FBS do not contain iron. Group 2 has grossly elevated iron by design. Group 4 comprised the iron-deficient group brought back to a normal level through the use of FAC. So the intention was to have iron levels roughly in the order $3 < 1 = 4 < 2$. Nonheme and intracellular iron levels were measured and are given in Table A.3.2.

There are four experimental groups and there are a number of reasonable group comparisons. It must be noted that there are a very large number of comparisons that could be made, each group versus one of the others, versus two or three of the others, each pair of two versus another two, etc. However, we present a standard shorthand for presenting group comparisons.

A.3.3   Methods of Analysis

For completeness and to orient people who are new to the area of analysis of microarray data, we have provided a high-level overview on the analysis flow in Table A.3.3. It must be kept in mind that the analysis strategy is still evolving in this

TABLE A.3.3:   Steps in the process of an analysis strategy for a microarray data set.

Step	Name	Description
1	Normalization	Adjust data values within a sample to a common mean or medial level
2	Quality control	Remove bad samples
3	Gene filtering	Remove unwanted genes, see Table A.3.5
4	Gene selection	Analysis of variance. Select genes with high signal to noise It is useful in formulating questions into linear contrasts
5	Clustering	Pattern finding among the selected genes Hierarchical clustering PCA (singular value decomposition) NMF, nonnegative matrix factorization
6	List processing	Gene ontology analysis Pathway analysis

TABLE A.3.4:　References for standard statistical analysis methods.

Analysis Method	Description
t-test	Statistical comparison between two groups http://en.wikipedia.org/wiki/T-test
Linear contrast	Use to compare a linear relationship among two or more groups http://en.wikipedia.org/wiki/Contrast_(statistics)
ANOVA	Analysis of variance, apportioning variance across different sources http://en.wikipedia.org/wiki/Analysis_of_variance
Clustering	Grouping similar objects together http://en.wikipedia.org/wiki/Data_clustering
SVD (PCA)	Singular value decomposition, matrix factorization (principal component analysis). See Good (1969) and Liu et al. (2003).
NMF	Nonnegative matrix factorization http://en.wikipedia.org/wiki/Nonnegative_matrix_factorization

area of complex experimentation. Data sets from GEO are normalized and hence, we omit that step in this reanalysis of CTM.

Again for orientation, we have listed the typical analysis methods used in microarray analysis in Table A.3.4. For most of these methods, there are good descriptions in the Wikipedia. For other methods, we refer to the introductory literature. Statistical methods used for the analysis of microarray data are largely conventional; the complication is that there are numerous methods, and different methods are used at different stages within the overall analysis strategy. We have omitted methods for the processing of the raw signals, as the data set we used were already processed and is available for analysis from GEO.

A hallmark of microarray analysis is the very large number of probe sets (genes). It is useful to filter the gene list to progressively smaller sets. For example, there are often control genes on a chip that are used in internal calibrations. These DNA sequence can come from entirely different species from those under consideration. Table A.3.5 gives a list of typical filtering operations. In any particular analysis, not

TABLE A.3.5:　Filtering steps for use in analysis of microarray data.

Step Number	Description of Filter
0	Starting number of genes
1	Control genes removed and all genes not from the species under consideration
2	Unexpressed and missing genes removed
3	Outliers samples removed
4	Low expression-level genes removed
5	ANOVA used to select treatment-related genes
6	Exclude low fold-change genes
7	Exclude duplicate probe sets (genes)

TABLE A.3.6: Model 2×2 factorial table—CTM experiment.

	Iron	
	No Added	
Media	**Iron**	**Added Iron**
DMEN + FBS	1	2 (hemin)
IMDM + Factors	3	4 (FAC)

all filtering steps will be used. Somewhat unconventionally, we list the statistical method, analysis of variance (ANOVA), as a filtering step. In experiments where there is only one outcome of interest, ANOVA would be listed as the statistical analysis step. For microarray data, it is better to think in terms of an analysis strategy (Table A.3.3).

It is worth presenting linear contrasts in some detail, leading to a clearer understanding on how to set up an experiment and analyze the results. If there are only two groups in the experiment, then the Contrast = (+1–1) is used as a shorthand for the comparison of group 1 with group 2. By definition, for a contrast, the sum of the coefficients must add to zero. If there are multiple groups, then a set of contrasts can be used as a shorthand for indicating the comparisons of interest and the nature of the calculations to be done. Consider a model 2×2 table (see Table A.3.6).

There are four groups.

	Group				
	1	2	3	4	Description
Contrast 1	(+1	+1	−1	−1)	Factor 1, Level 1 versus Level 2
Contrast 2	(+1	−1	+1	−1)	Factor 2, Level 1 versus Level 2
Contrast 3	(+1	−1	−1	+1)	Interaction of Factors 1 and 2

In the next section of the paper, Analysis, we will provide a set of contrasts used for the analysis of the CTM data set and it may be useful to look ahead (see Table A.3.7).

Principal components analysis (PCA), is quite popular for analyzing the micro array data. The mathematical matrix-factorization method and singular value decomposition are the bases of PCA (see Figure A.3.2). A matrix X is factored into two matrices, W and H. In these two matrices, we attempt to capture the signal in the data set. The diagonal matrix Λ is a matrix of singular values, scaling factors, that gives the importance of the vectors that make up W and H. What is not captured in $W\Lambda H$ is the noise of the system. If the elements of X are all positive or zero, then the factorization can be computed using a nonnegative matrix factorization, NMF, where the elements of W and H are also all positive or zero. The NMF appears to be quite useful for microarray data (Kim and Tidor, 2003; Brunet et al., 2004; Fogel et al., 2006). The NMF has the alleged useful property that states that separate mechanisms go for separate vectors of W and H (Donoho and Stodden 2004; Lee and Seung, 1999).

TABLE A.3.7:   Contrasts of interest in our analysis.

Contrast	Group 1 (DMEM)	Group 2 (DMEM) +Hemin)	Group 3 (IMDM)	Group 4 (IMDM) +FAC)	Contrast Description
Contrast 1	-1	1	0	0	High iron versus normal iron (in medium DMEM)
Contrast 2	0	0	1	-1	Low iron versus normal iron (in medium IMDM)
Contrast 3	-1	1	-1	1	Low ferritin versus high ferritin
Contrast 4	-1	0	0	1	Normal iron (in DMEM) versus normal iron (in IMDM)
Contrast 5	0	1	0	-1	High iron (in DMEM) versus normal iron (in IMDM)

$$X = W \Lambda H + N$$

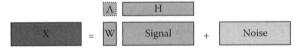

FIGURE A.3.2:   Matrix-factorization using a singular-value decomposition.

A.3.4   Analysis

We would not discuss normalization, as the data from GEO are already normalized. The CTM filtered out some genes (any gene with the annotation "ignore") before making a deposit to GEO. Therefore, we removed any genes noted as control genes, positive or negative. We then checked whether any remaining gene contained the term "homo sapiens" or "HS". The filtered gene counts are given in Table A.3.8.

As a quality control step (Table A.3.3, Step 2), we computed a PCA analysis of the intensity data (Figure A.3.3) and ensured that no samples were outside the 95%

TABLE A.3.8:   Filtering of gene list: part 1—preprocessing.

Original	Remove Ctrl_Type = Ignore*	Remove Ctrl_Type = Pos|Neg	Select Genes of *Homo sapiens*
22575	22153	21073	20865

*   The data downloaded from GEO Web site is the one after this step.

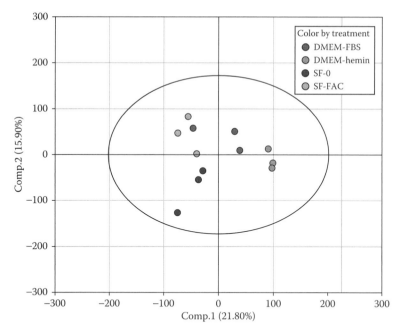

FIGURE A.3.3:   QC plot of the first and second PCA scores for the 12 samples.

confidence ellipse. We observed no chips to be outliers. The CTM removed one sample as an outlier. Careful examination of clustering the samples and examination of the correlations of the genes from one chip to another can be employed to support their decision.

Consequently, we constructed linear contrasts (Table A.3.3, Step 4) that address the questions at issue. It can be observed from Table A.3.7 along with Table A.3.6 that Contrasts 1–3 are those given in CTM. The first two contrasts are relatively clean in that only one major factor differs between the two groups being compared. Contrast 3 is more problematic in that there is both a difference in iron level and media. As the IMDM media was constructed to be semisynthetic, there could be rather profound differences between this medium and the DMEN medium. We added two additional contrasts to show how contrasts are used to focus on questions and also to show the difficulties of confounding experimental conditions. Contrast 4 tests for a general media effect. The comparison is not balanced for iron effects; hence, the results could be misleading. Contrast 5 tests for normal versus high iron, but the two treatments are with different media and hence, there is a confounding of media effects with iron effect. In the discussion section, we discuss an alternative experimental design (see Table A.3.9 that is more balanced).

The statistical filtering, ANOVA, is executed (Table A.3.3, Step 4). Performing ANOVA on 20,865 genes means that we need to adjust the analysis for multiple testing. It is common to use the false discovery rate (FDR) adjustment of Benjamini and Hochberg (1995). We set the level at 0.10, and so we expected 10% of our claims

TABLE A.3.9: Model
2 × 2 factorial table.

	Iron	
Media	**Normal**	**Elevated**
DMEM	1	2
IMDM	4	5*

* New treatment, IMDM media
with excess iron.

TABLE A.3.10: Filtering of gene list. ANOVA on 20865 probe sets.

Contrast	Alpha = 0.1 (FDR)	Alpha = 0.1 (FDR) and FC >1.5	Remove Duplicates
Contrast 1	744	91	78
Contrast 2	349	50	45
Contrast 3	498	162	149
Contrast 4	401	69	62
Contrast 5	1467	420	362

TABLE A.3.11: Merging of gene lists for all contrasts.

Total of C1 to C5 List	Remove Probe Sets with Same ID	Remove Duplicate Genes
696	539	535

to be false positives. We subsequently removed any genes where the fold-change was less than 1.50. Finally, we removed the duplicate genes. (It is common for chip manufacturers to place duplicate genes on their chips. Some of these will be significantly changed. These need to be removed to make a nonredundant list.) Table A.3.10 gives the gene counts for this filtering for each of the five contrasts. Table A.3.11 merges the significant genes over the five contrasts and removes the duplicate genes with the same probe-set ID or the same gene name. It is interesting to note which genes are changed in common with respect to the contrasts of interest. Figure A.3.4 gives the Venn diagram for contrasts 1–2, the contrasts used by CTM along with the results for contrast 3, which gives genes associated with an increase in iron. Figure A.3.5 gives the Venn diagram for contrasts 1, 4, and 5. It is intriguing that the results given in these Venn diagrams can be related to the confounding in the experiment.

Figure A.3.6 gives the rather standard hierarchical clustering of the significant genes (rows) and samples (columns) of Table A.3.3, Step 5a. The high iron, group 2, DMEM-hemin, green in the figure and the normal iron, group 4, IMDM-FAC, yellow in the figure, are rather cleanly clustered. The normal iron group, group 1, DMEM-FBS, blue in the figure, is split. This result is awkward and might have probably led CTM to remove one sample. It is natural to consider the clustering of the samples

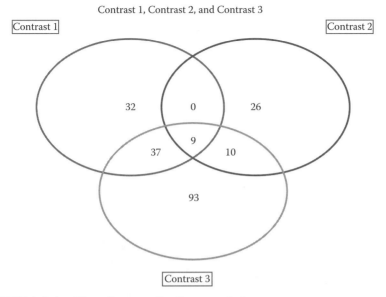

FIGURE A.3.4: Venn diagrams for Contrasts 1–3.

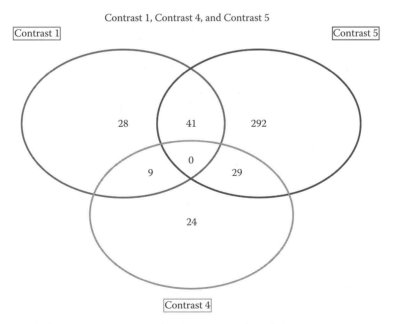

FIGURE A.3.5: Venn diagrams for Contrasts 1, 4, and 5.

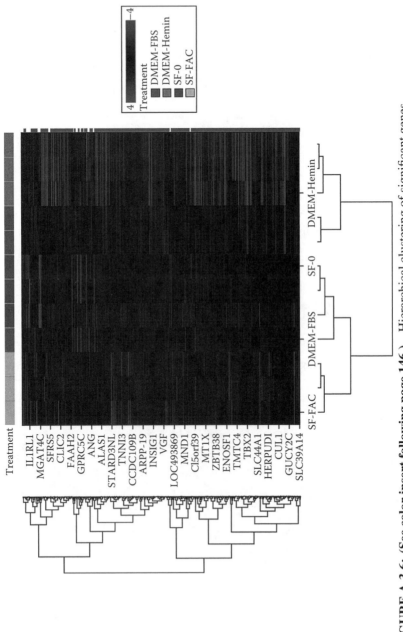

FIGURE A.3.6: (See color insert following page 146.)   Hierarchical clustering of significant genes.

first, as a clean separation of the samples implies that the ANOVA selected genes are up to the task of making sense of the data.

We considered two other clustering methods and presented the result for NMF in Figure A.3.7 a through c. It can be observed that groups 2 and 4 are cleanly separated, while groups 1 and 3 are put together, just as in hierarchical clustering. The gene weights, H (not given here) in the matrix factorization, as shown in Figure A.3.2, are potentially quite useful. Often in NMF many of the weights are very close to zero and the genes with the remaining positive weights are the important genes for the factorization.

A.3.4.1 Discussion

The CTM commented that body-iron homeostasis is strictly regulated, with three described regulators controlling the iron absorption; whereas, excretion is not regulated. We might expect the clustering, matrix factorization, and significant genes to point to these three mechanisms. Furthermore, there are four rather distinct treatments that point to finding four clusters/mechanisms. Calibration of treatments can be problematic; if the treatments are too severe, then the secondary reactions can occur and multiple mechanisms may be evoked. When two experimental factors are confounded, for example, media and iron levels, it is not possible to point to one factor or the other with assurance.

Balanced factorial designs are very popular in many areas of applied science, because they increase the number of questions that can be asked with the same amount of experimental material. A complicating factor in this paper is the confounding of experimental procedures with the questions at issue. Consider a hypothetical experiment given in Table A.3.9. There are two factors, media and iron level and each is at two levels. The DMEN and IMDM are supplemented with two levels of iron, low and normal. So now, the contrasts $(-1\ -1\ 1\ 1)$ and $(-1\ 1\ -1\ 1)$ present what are called "main effect" for the media and iron level, and both these contrasts use all the data. The sample size is effectively doubled. Of course, the new experiment does not address the effect in the case of iron deficit, but it does address the normal versus high iron (the iron overload case) in a more statistically powerful way. Two questions are asked for the price of one, which is a good deal.

The NCBI GEO database is a very valuable resource. The obvious utility is to obviate the need for an experiment. The fact that the data is freely available means that you do not have to trust the analysis of the original experimenters; you can do the analysis yourself. If you chose to replicate the experiment, then you have the data to confirm or deny your claims. We think these data sets have a great utility for training in the analysis of these complex microarray experiments. Having a data set with a literature paper gives you a benchmark to evaluate your own analysis. With good software, the reanalysis is reasonably fast and different analysis strategies can be employed. Each step of Table A.3.3 has various alternatives. Also, certain combinations of methods may be better than the others. For example, use of some method of variable selection prior to ANOVA would be advantageous. Any method

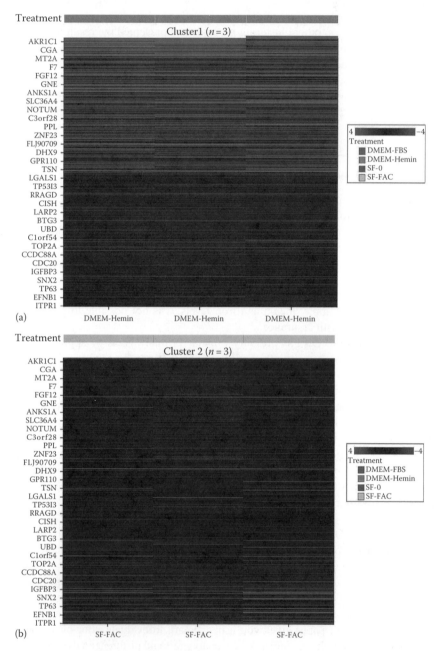

(a)

(b)

FIGURE A.3.7: (See color insert following page 146.)   (a) NMF, cluster 1, group 2, high iron (hemin), (b) NMF, cluster 2, group 4, normal iron (FAC).

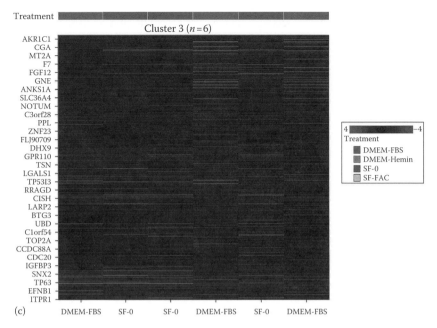

FIGURE A.3.7: (continued) (See color insert following page 146.) (c) NMF, cluster 3, groups 1 and 3.

that removes genes before statistical testing should increase the ability to determine the real effects.

A.3.5   Data and Software

The data used in this article can be found at http://www.ncbi.nlm.nih.gov/geo/ and searched using the experiment name GSE3573.

The microarray analysis software used in this article can be found at www.omicsoft. com, along with detailed tutorials on the use of the software. The free program BioNMF, www.dacya.ucm.es/apascual/bioNMF, can be used for NMF.

References (for Appendix)

Benjamini, Y. and Hochberg, Y. 1995. Controlling the false discovery rate: a practical and powerful approach to multiple testing. *J. R. Stat. Soc.* B 57, 289–300.

Brunet, J.P., Tamayo, P., Golub, T.R., and Mesirov, J.P. 2004. Metagenes and molecular pattern discovery using matrix factorization. *Proc. Natl. Acad. Sci. U S A* 101, 4164–4169.

Chicault, C., Toutain, B., Monnier, A., Aubry, M. et al. 2006. Iron-related transcriptomic variations in CaCo-2 cells, an in vitro model of intestinal absorptive cells. *Physiol. Genomics* 26, 55–67.

Donoho, D. and Stodden, V. 2004. When does non-negative matrix factorization give a correct decomposition into parts? *Advances in Neural Information Processing Systems* 17.

Fogel, P., Young, S.S., Hawkins, D.M., and Ledirac, N. 2006. Inferential, robust non-negative matrix factorization analysis of microarray data. *Bioinformatics* 23, 44–49.

Good, I.J. 1969. Some applications of the singular decomposition of a matrix. *Technometrics* 11, 823–831.

Kim, P.M. and Tidor, B. 2003. Subsystem identification through dimensionality reduction of large-scale gene expression data. *Genome Res.* 13, 1706–1718.

Lee, D.D. and Seung, H.S. 1999. Learning the parts of objects by non-negative matrix factorization. *Nature* 401, 788–791.

Liu, L., Hawkins, D.M., Ghosh, S., and Young, S.S. 2003. Robust singular value decomposition analysis of microarray data. *Proc. Natl. Acad. Sci. U S A* 100, 13167–13172.

Wheeler, D.L., Barrett, T., Benson, D.A., Bryant, S.H., et al. 2007. Database resources of the National Center for Biotechnology Information. *Nucleic Acids Res.* 35, D5–D12.

3.6   Some Further Statistical Considerations

Statistical process plays an important role in translational research and TM. In this book, we define a statistical process of translational research and TM as a translational process for (1) determining the association between some independent parameters observed in one research area (e.g., basic research, such as early discoveries, nonclinical research, and preclinical research) and a dependent variable observed from another research area (e.g., first-in-human clinical research); (2) establishing a predictive model between the independent parameters and the dependent response variable; and (3) validating the established predictive model. As an example, in animal studies for pharmaceutical R&D, the independent variables may include *in vitro* assay results, pharmacological activities, such as pharmacokinetics and pharmacodynamics, as well as dose toxicities, and the dependent variable could be the clinical outcomes. It must be noted that a statistical process is often employed to calibrate an instrument, such as a gas chromatograph (GC), HPLC, or a radioimmunoassay (RIA), which is usually employed in assay development for a newly developed compound in early drug discovery. A brief description on the model selection/validation for establishment of a predictive model, tests for one-way and two-way translational process, statistical evaluation on whether an animal model can be predictive of a human model, translations among various study endpoints in clinical trials, and the use of clinical trial simulation are provided in the following sections.

3.7   Model Selection and Validation

When a new pharmaceutical compound is discovered, analytical methods or test procedures are necessarily developed for determining the active ingredients of the compound in compliance with USP/NF standards for the identity, strength, quality, purity, stability, and reproducibility of the compound. An analytical method or test procedure is usually developed, based on instruments such as HPLC. Current good manufacturing practices (CGMP) indicates that an instrument must be suitable for its intended purposes and be capable of producing valid results with certain degrees of accuracy and reliability. Therefore, the instrument must be calibrated, inspected, and checked routinely according to written procedures. As a result, instrument calibration is essential to meet the established written procedures or specifications.

A typical approach to instrument calibration is to have a number of known standard-concentration preparations put through the instrument, to obtain the corresponding responses. Based on these standard-concentration preparations and their corresponding responses, an estimated calibration curve (or standard curve) can be obtained by fitting an appropriate statistical model between the standard-concentration preparations and their corresponding responses. The fitted regression model for the calibration curve is required to be validated for accuracy and reliability. For a given sample, the validated calibration curve (or standard curve) can then be used to quantitate the concentration of the given sample. As indicated by the USP/NF, the validation of an analytical method or a test procedure can be carried out by assessing a set of performance characteristics or analytical validation parameters. These validation parameters include, but are not limited to, accuracy, precision, linearity, range, specificity, LOD, limit of quantitation (LOQ), and ruggedness. More details regarding the calibration process of an analytical method or a testing procedure, model selection, and validation of the established model are presented in Chapter 4.

3.8   Tests for Translational Process

In practice, it is important to ensure that the translational process is accurate and reliable with certain statistical assurance. One of the statistical criteria is to examine the closeness between the observed response and the predicted response by the translational process. To study this, we denote the independent and the dependent variable in the translational process by x and y, respectively. In practice, we would first study the association between x and y and then build up a model. Subsequently, the model is validated based on some criteria. For simplicity, we can assume that x and y can be described by the following linear model:

$$y = a + bx + e$$

where e follows a distribution with mean 0 and variance σ_e^2. Then, from the above-mentioned model, the normality assumptions a and b can be estimated. Thus, we have established the following relationship:

$$y = \hat{a} + \hat{b}x$$

Traditionally, the closeness of an observed y and its predicted value $\hat{y}$ obtained based on the above-fitted regression model was considered. In other words, it is desirable to have a high probability that the relative difference between y and $\hat{y}$ is lesser than a clinically or scientifically meaningful difference (say δ), i.e., the probability

$$p = P\left\{\left|\frac{y - \hat{y}}{y}\right| < \delta\right\}$$

needs to be relatively high. Thus, it is of interest to test the following hypotheses:

$$H_0: p \leq p_0 \quad \text{versus} \quad H_a: p > p_0$$

where p_0 is a predetermined desirable probability. The idea is to reject H_0 and favor H_a. In other words, we would like to reject the null hypothesis and conclude that the established translational model is validated. Under the null hypothesis, Chow (2006) derived a test based on the maximum likelihood estimate of p. It must be noted that the above translational process is usually referred to as a one-way translational process in TM. In other words, as an example, the one-way translational process in pharmaceutical development translates the early discoveries of basic research to the clinical results. As indicated by Pizzo (2006), the translational process should be a two-way translation process. In other words, a two-way translational process translates the clinical results back to basic research discoveries. In this case, we can exchange x and y, and consider the following model:

$$x = c + dy + \varepsilon$$

Consequently, we have another predictive model

$$x = \hat{c} + \hat{d}y$$

Now, the idea for the validation of a two-way translational process can be described as follows:

> **Step 1:** For a given set of data (x,y), established a predictive model. In other words, determine
> $$f(x)$$

> **Step 2:** Evaluate the one-way closeness between y and $\hat{y}$ based on a test for $H_0: p \leq p_0$ versus $H_a: p > p_0$.
> Proceed to the next step if the one-way translational process is validated.

> **Step 3:** Consider $\hat{y}$ as the observed y and obtain the predicted value of x, i.e., $\hat{x}$ based on the established model between x and y (i.e., $x = g(y)$). Note that in the above example, $x = c + dy + \varepsilon$.

> **Step 4:** Evaluate the one-way closeness between x and $\hat{x}$ based on a test for $H_0: p \leq p_0$ versus $H_a: p > p_0$, where

$$p = P\left\{\left|\frac{y - \hat{y}}{y}\right| < \delta \quad \text{and} \quad \left|\frac{x - \hat{x}}{x}\right| < \Delta\right\}$$

To test for a two-way translation, consider the hypotheses given in Step 2 that H_0: $p \leq p_0$ versus H_a: $p > p_0$. The idea is to reject H_0 and favor H_a.

It must be noted that since we only consider relative changes, the difference between δ and Δ is considered the degree of lost in translation. Ideally, δ should be equal to Δ. If it is easy to derive a test, we can assume that $\delta = \Delta$. In fact, it will be a good idea to also derive a test for the null hypothesis that $\delta = \Delta$. To test the two-way translation, consider the following hypotheses:

$$H_0: p \leq p_0 \quad \text{versus} \quad H_a: p > p_0$$

The idea is to reject H_0 and favor H_a. In other words, we would like to reject the null hypothesis and conclude that the established one is validated. With respect to the null hypothesis, following the idea described in Chow (2006), a test for two-way translational process can be similarly obtained.

3.9 Animal Model versus Human Model

In TM, a common question is that whether an animal model is predictive of a human model. To address this question, in addition to tests for one-way and two-way translation, one may consider the following test for similarity between an animal model and a human model. For illustration purpose, we will only consider the one-way translation. Let $y = \hat{a} + \hat{b}x$ be the predictive model obtained from the one-way translational process, based on data from an animal population. Thus, a given x_0, $y = \hat{a} + \hat{b}x_0$ follows a distribution with mean μ_y and variance σ_y^2 under the animal population. The animal population is denoted by $(\mu_{animal}, \sigma_{animal})$, where $\mu_{animal} = \mu_y$ and $\sigma_{animal} = \sigma_y$. Assuming that the linear relationship between x and y can be applied to a human population, it is expected that y will follow a distribution with mean $\mu_y + \varepsilon$ and variance $C\sigma_y$. The effect size adjusted for standard deviation under the human population is then given by

$$\left| \frac{\mu_{human}}{\sigma_{human}} \right| = \left| \frac{\mu_y + \varepsilon}{C\sigma_y} \right| = |\Delta| \left| \frac{\mu_y}{\sigma_y} \right| = |\Delta| \left| \frac{\mu_{animal}}{\sigma_{animal}} \right|$$

where

$$\Delta = \frac{1 + \varepsilon/\mu_y}{C}$$

Chow et al. (2002) referred to Δ as a sensitivity index when changing from a target population to another. The effect size under the human population is inflated (or reduced) by the factor of Δ, and is usually referred to as the sensitivity index. If $\varepsilon = 0$ and $C = 1$ (i.e., $\Delta = 1$), we then claim that the animal model is predictive of human model. Note that the shift and scale parameters (i.e., ε and C) can be estimated by

$$\hat{\varepsilon} = \hat{\mu}_{human} - \hat{\mu}_{animal}$$

and

$$\hat{C} = \hat{\sigma}_{\text{human}} / \hat{\sigma}_{\text{animal}}$$

respectively, where $(\hat{\mu}_{\text{animal}}, \hat{\sigma}_{\text{animal}})$ and $(\hat{\mu}_{\text{human}}, \hat{\sigma}_{\text{human}})$ are some estimates of (μ_y, σ_y) under the animal and the human population, respectively. As a result, the sensitivity index can be estimated by

$$\hat{\Delta} = \frac{1 + \hat{\varepsilon} / \hat{\mu}}{\hat{C}}$$

3.10 Translation among Study Endpoints

In clinical trials, it is not uncommon that a study is powered based on a primary study endpoint (e.g., absolute change from baseline), however, the collected data is analyzed based on a different study endpoint (e.g., percent change from baseline or the percentage of patients who show some improvement based on another parameter, such as absolute change from baseline). It is very controversial when interpreting the analysis results when a significant result is observed based on one study endpoint but not the other. For example, in some clinical studies for the evaluation of possible weight reduction of a test treatment in obese patients, the analysis and interpretation between the concept of absolute change and the concept of percent change (or the percentage of patients who have a desired absolute change) are very different. In practice, it is then of interest to explore how an observed significant absolute change can be translated to a percent change or a percentage of patients who will show an improvement, based on the absolute change. An immediate impact is the power analysis for sample-size calculation. The sample size required to achieve the desired power, based on the absolute change could be very different from that obtained based on the percent change (or the percentage of patients who show an improvement based on the absolute change) at the α level of significance.

Let x and y be the observed absolute change and the percent change, respectively, of a primary study endpoint (e.g., body weight) of a given clinical trial. Thus, the hypotheses of interest based on the absolute change are given by

$$H_{01}: \mu_x = 0 \quad \text{versus} \quad H_{a1}: \mu_x = \delta$$

where δ is the difference of clinical importance. For the percent change, the hypotheses of interest are given by

$$H_{02}: \mu_y = 0 \quad \text{versus} \quad H_{a2}: \mu_y = \Delta$$

where Δ is the difference of clinical importance. In practice, the clinical equivalent value of δ to Δ is not known. For a better understanding, Figures 1.5.1 and 1.5.2 illustrate (1) plots of δ and Δ versus n (sample size) for a fixed desired power and (2) plots δ and Δ versus power for a fixed sample size n, respectively. In addition, if we consider a patient as a responder, if his/her absolute change of the primary study endpoint is greater than δ, then it is of interest to test the following hypotheses:

$$H_{03}: p_x = \eta \quad \text{versus} \quad H_{a3}: p_x > \eta$$

where p_x is the proportion of patients whose absolute change of the primary study endpoint is greater than δ. In practice, we may claim superiority (clinically) of the test treatment, if we reject the null hypothesis at $\eta = 50\%$ and favor the alternative hypothesis that $p_x > 50\%$. However, this lacks statistical justification. For a non-inferiority (or superiority) trial, how the selection of a non-inferiority margin of μ_x can be translated to the non-inferiority margin of p_x must be determined.

3.11 Trial Simulation

Clinical trial simulation is a process that uses computers to mimic the conduct of a study by creating virtual subjects (experimental units) and extrapolate (or predict) outcomes for each virtual subject based on the prespecified models. The primary objective of trial simulation is multifold. First, it is to monitor the conduct of the trial, project outcomes, anticipate problems, and recommend remedies before it is too late. Second, it is to extrapolate (or predict) the outcomes beyond the scope of previous studies from which the existing models were derived using the model techniques. Third, it is to study the validity and robustness of the trial under various assumptions of the study designs. Trial simulation is often conducted to verify (or confirm) the models depicting the relationships between the inputs, such as dose, dosing time, subject characteristics, and disease severity and the outcomes, such as changes in the signs and symptoms or adverse events within the study domain in discovery and clinical TM. In practice, trial simulation is often considered to predict potential outcomes under different assumptions and various design scenarios at the planning stage of a trial for a better planning of the actual trial.

Trial simulation is a powerful tool in pharmaceutical development. The concept of trial simulation is very intuitive and easy to implement. In practice, trial simulation is often considered as a useful tool for the evaluation of the performance of a test treatment under a model with complicated situations. It can achieve the goal with minimum assumptions by controlling Type I error rate, effectively. It can also be used to visualize the dynamic trial process from patient recruitment, drug distribution, treatment administration, and pharmacokinetic processes to biomarker development and clinical responses. In this chapter, we will review the application of clinical trial simulations in both the early and late phases of pharmaceutical development.

The framework of trial simulation is rather simple. It consists of trial design, study objectives (hypotheses), model, and statistical tests. For the trial design, critical design features, such as (1) a parallel or crossover design, (2) a balanced or unbalanced design, (3) the number of treatment groups, and (4) algorithms, need to be clearly specified. Under the trial design, hypotheses, such as testing for equality, superiority, or non-inferiority/equivalence can then be formulated for achieving the study objectives. A statistical model is necessarily implemented to generate virtual subjects and extrapolate (or predict) the outcomes. With respect to the hypotheses, we can then evaluate the performance of the test treatment through the study of statistical properties of the statistical tests derived under the null and alternative hypotheses. More specifically, we begin a trial simulation by choosing a statistical model under a valid trial design with various assumptions according to the trial setting. We then simulate the trial by creating virtual subjects and generating the outcomes for each virtual subject, based on the model specifications under the null hypothesis for a large number of times (say m times). For each simulation carried out, we calculate the test statistics. The m-test statistic values constitute a distribution of the test statistics numerically. Similarly, we repeat the process to simulate the trial under the alternative hypothesis for m times. The m-test statistic values obtained represent the distribution of the test statistic under the alternative hypothesis. These two distributions can be used to determine the critical region for a given α level of significance, p-value for a given data, and the corresponding power for the given critical region.

It must be noted that the computer simulation starts with generating data under the null hypothesis. The data is often generated from a simple distribution, such as a normal distribution for continuous variables, a binary distribution for discrete variables, and an exponential distribution for time-to-event data. The generation of simulated data occurs only once per simulation carried out. More details regarding the computer-trial simulation will be further discussed in Chapter 4.

References

Chow, S.C. 2006. Statistical tests in translational medicine. Technical report, Department of Biostatistics and Bioinformatics, Duke University School of Medicine, Durham, North Carolina.

Chow, S.C., Shao, J., and Hu, O.Y.P. 2002. Assessing sensitivity and similarity in bridging studies. *Journal of Biopharmaceutical Statistics* 12, 385–400.

Pizzo, P.A. 2006. The Dean's Newsletter. Stanford University School of Medicine, Stanford, California.

Shih, W.J. 2001. Clinical trials for drug registrations in Asian Pacific countries: Proposal for a new paradigm from a statistical perspective. *Controlled Clinical Trials* 22, 357–366.

USP/NF 2000. The XXIV and the National Formulary XIX. The United States Pharmacopedial Convention, Rockville, Maryland.

Chapter 4

Biomarker Development

Mark Chang

Contents

4.1 Introduction

As indicated by Pizzo (2006), translational medicine (TM) can have a much broader definition, referring to the development and application of new technologies, biomedical devices, and therapies in a patient-driven environment such as clinical trials, where the emphasis is on early patient testing and evaluation. Thus, in this chapter, our emphasis will be placed on biomarker development in early clinical development. Since biomarker development is often carried out under an adaptive design setting in early clinical development, we will focus on statistical consideration for the use of biomarker-adaptive design in early clinical development for TM.

Biomarkers, when compared with a true endpoint such as survival, can often be measured earlier, easily, and more frequently, are less subject to competing risks, and less confounded. The utilization of biomarker will lead to a better target population with a larger effect size, a smaller sample-size required, and faster decision-making.

With the advancement of proteomic, genomic, and genetic technologies, personalized medicine with the right drug for the right patient has become possible.

Conley and Taube (2004) described the future of biomarker/genomic markers in cancer therapy: "The elucidation of the human genome and fifty years of biological studies have laid the groundwork for a more informed method for treating cancer with the prospect of realizing improved survival. Advanced in knowledge about the molecular abnormalities, signaling pathways, influence the local tissue milieu and the relevance of genetic polymorphism offer hope of designing effective therapies tailored for a given cancer in particular individual, as well as the possibility of avoiding unnecessary toxicity."

Wang et al. (2006) from FDA have pointed out: "Generally, when the primary clinical efficacy outcome in a phase III trial requires much longer time to observe, a surrogate endpoint thought to be strongly associated with the clinical endpoint may be chosen as the primary efficacy variable in phase II trials. The results of the phase II studies then provide an estimated effect size on the surrogate endpoint, which is supposedly able to help size the phase III trial for the primary clinical efficacy endpoint, where often it is thought to have a smaller effect size."

What exactly is a biomarker? National Institutes of Health Workshop (De Gruttola, 2001) gave the following definitions. *Biomarker* is a characteristic that is objectively measured and evaluated as an indicator of normal biologic processes, pathogenic processes, or pharmacological responses to a therapeutic intervention. *Clinical endpoint* (or outcome) is a characteristic or variable that reflects how a patient feels or functions, or how long a patient survives. *Surrogate endpoint* is a biomarker intended to substitute for a clinical endpoint. Biomarkers can also be classified as classifier, prognostic, and predictive biomarkers.

Classifier biomarker is a marker, e.g., a DNA marker, that usually does not change over the course of the study. A classifier biomarker can be used to select the most appropriate target population or even for personalized treatment. For example, a study drug is expected to have effects on a population with a biomarker, which is only 20% of the overall patient population. Because the sponsor suspects that the drug may not work for the overall patient population, it may be efficient and ethical to run a trial only for the subpopulations with the biomarker rather than the general patient population. On the other hand, some biomarkers such as RNA markers are expected to change over the course of the study. This type of marker can be either a prognostic or a predictive marker.

Prognostic biomarker informs about the clinical outcomes, independent of treatment. It provides information about natural course of the disease in an individual with or without treatment under study. A prognostic marker does not inform the effect of the treatment. For example, NSCLC patients receiving either EGFR inhibitors or chemotherapy have better outcomes with a mutation than without it. Prognostic markers can be used to separate good and poor prognosis patients at the time of diagnosis. If expression of the marker clearly separates patients with an excellent prognosis from those with a poor prognosis, then the marker can be used to aid the decision about how aggressive the therapy needs to be. The poor prognosis patients might be considered for clinical trials of novel therapies that will, hopefully, be more effective (Conley and Taube, 2004). Prognostic markers may also inform the possible mechanisms responsible for the poor prognosis, thus leading to the identification of new targets for treatment and new effective therapeutics.

Predictive biomarker informs about the treatment effect on the clinical endpoint. A predictive marker can be population-specific: a marker can be predictive for population A but not for population B. A predictive biomarker, when compared with true endpoints like survival, can often be measured earlier, easily, and more frequently and is less subject to competing risks. For example, in a trial of a cholesterol-lowering drug, the ideal endpoint may be death or development of coronary artery disease (CAD). However, such a study usually requires thousands of patients and many years to conduct. Therefore, it is desirable to have a biomarker, such as a reduction in post-treatment cholesterol, if it predicts the reductions in the incidence of CAD. Another example would be an oncology study where the ultimate endpoint is death. However, when a patient has disease progression, the physician will switch the patient's initial treatment to an alternative treatment. Such treatment modalities will jeopardize the assessment of treatment effect on survival because the treatment switching is response-adaptive rather than random. If a marker, such as time-to-progression (TTP) or response rate (RR), is used as the primary endpoint, then we will have much cleaner efficacy assessments because the biomarker assessment is performed before the treatment switching occurs.

In this chapter, we will discuss adaptive designs using classifier, prognosis, and predictive markers.

4.2 Design with Classifier Biomarker

4.2.1 Setting the Scene

As mentioned earlier, a drug might have different effects in different patient populations. A hypothetical case is presented in Table 4.1, where RR_+ and RR_- are the response rates for biomarker-positive population (BPP) and biomarker-negative population (BNP), respectively. In the example, there is a treatment effect of 25% in the 10 million patient population with the biomarker, but only 9% in the 50 million general patient population. The sponsor faces the dilemma of whether to target the general patient population or use biomarkers to select a smaller set of patients that are expected to have a bigger response to the drug.

TABLE 4.1: Response rate and sample-size required.

	Population	$RR_+\%$	$RR_-\%$	Sample-Size
Biomarker (+)	10M	50	25	160*
Biomarker (−)	40M	30	25	
Total	50M	34	25	1800

* 800 subjects screened. Power = 80%.

There are several challenges: (1) the estimated effect size for each subpopulation at the design stage is often very inaccurate; (2) a cost is associated with screening patients for the biomarker; (3) the test for detecting the biomarker often requires a high sensitivity and specificity, and the screening tool may not be available at the time of the clinical trial; and (4) screening patients for the biomarker may cause a burden and impact patient recruitment. These factors must be considered in the design.

4.2.2 Classic Design with Classifier Biomarker

Denote treatment difference between the test and control groups by δ_+, δ_-, and δ, for biomarker-positive, biomarker-negative, and overall patient populations, respectively. The null hypothesis for biomarker-positive subpopulation is

$$H_{01}: \delta_+ = 0. \tag{4.1}$$

The null hypothesis for biomarker-negative subpopulation is

$$H_{02}: \delta_- = 0. \tag{4.2}$$

The null hypothesis for overall population is

$$H_0: \delta = 0. \tag{4.3}$$

Without loss of generality, assume that the first n patients have the biomarker among N patients and the test statistic for the subpopulation is given by

$$Z_+ = \frac{\sum_{i=1}^{n} x_i - \sum_{i=1}^{n} y_i}{n\sigma} \sqrt{\frac{n}{2}} \sim N(0,1) \text{ under } H_0, \tag{4.4}$$

where x_i and y_i $(i = 1,\ldots,n)$ are the responses in treatments A and B.

Similarly, the test statistic for biomarker-negative group is defined as

$$Z_- = \frac{\left(\sum_{i=n+1}^{N} x_i - \sum_{i=n+1}^{N} y_i\right)}{(N-n)\sigma} \sqrt{\frac{N-n}{2}} \sim N(0,1) \text{ under } H_0. \tag{4.5}$$

The test statistic for overall population is given by

$$Z = \frac{\hat{\delta}}{\sigma} \sqrt{\frac{N}{2}} = T_+ \sqrt{\frac{n}{N}} + T_- \sqrt{\frac{N-n}{N}} \sim N(0,1) \text{ under } H_0. \tag{4.6}$$

We choose the test statistic for the trial as

$$T = \max(Z, Z_+). \tag{4.7}$$

It can be shown that the correlation coefficient between Z and Z_+ is

$$\rho = \sqrt{\frac{n}{N}}. \tag{4.8}$$

Therefore, the stopping boundary can be determined by

$$\Pr\left(T \geq z_{2,1-\alpha}|H_o\right) = \alpha, \tag{4.9}$$

where $z_{2,1-\alpha}$ is the bivariate normal $100(1-\alpha)$-equipercentage point under H_o.
The p-value corresponding to an observed test statistic t is given by

$$p = \Pr\left(T \geq t|H_o\right). \tag{4.10}$$

The power can be calculated using

$$\Pr\left(T \geq z_{2,1-\alpha}|H_a\right) = \alpha. \tag{4.11}$$

The numerical integration or simulations can be performed to evaluate $z_{2,1-\alpha}$ and the power.

Note that the test statistic for the overall population can be defined as

$$Z = w_1 Z_+ + w_2 Z_-,$$

where w_1 and w_2 are constants satisfying $w_1^2 + w_2^2 = 1$. In such a case, the correlation coefficient between Z and Z_+ is $\rho = w_1$.

More generally, if there are m groups under consideration, we can define a statistic for the gth group as

$$Z_g = \frac{\hat{\delta}_g}{\sigma}\sqrt{\frac{n_g}{2}} \sim N(0,1) \text{ under } H_o. \tag{4.12}$$

The test statistic for the overall population is given by

$$T = \max\left\{Z_1,...,Z_g\right\}, \tag{4.13}$$

where $\{Z_1,...,Z_m\}$ is asymptotically m-variate standard normal distribution under H_o with expectation $\mathbf{0} = \{0,...,0\}$ and correlation matrix $\mathbf{R} = \{\rho_{ij}\}$. It can be easily shown that the correlation between Z_i and Z_j is given by

$$\rho_{ij} = \sqrt{\frac{n_{ij}}{n_i n_j}}, \tag{4.14}$$

where n_{ij} is the number of concordant pairs between the ith and jth groups.

The asymptotic formulation for power calculation with the multiple tests is similar to that for multiple-contrast tests (Bretz and Hothorn, 2002):

$$\Pr\left(T \geq z_{m,1-\alpha}|H_a\right)$$
$$= 1 - \Pr(Z_1 < z_{m,1-\alpha} \cap \cdots \cap T_m < z_{m,1-\alpha}|H_a$$
$$= 1 - \Phi_m\left((\mathbf{z}_{m,1-\alpha} - e)\operatorname{diag}\left(\frac{1}{v_0},...,\frac{1}{v_m}\right); \mathbf{0}; \mathbf{R}\right),$$

where $\mathbf{z}_{m,1-\alpha} = (z_{m,1-\alpha},...,z_{m,1-\alpha})$ stands for the m-variate normal $100(1-\alpha)$-equipercentage point under H_0, $\mathbf{e} = (E_a(T_0),...,E_a(T_m))$ and $\mathbf{v} = (v_0,...,v_m) = \left(\sqrt{V_0(T_0)},\sqrt{V_1(T_1)},...,\sqrt{V_1(T_m)}\right)$ are vectorially summarized expectations and standard errors.

The power is given by

$$p = \Pr(T \geq z_{m,1-p}). \tag{4.15}$$

For other types of endpoints, we can use inverse-normal method, i.e., $Z_g = \Phi(1-p_g)$ in Equation 4.12, where p_g is the p-value for the hypothesis test in the gth population group, then Equations 4.14 and 4.15 are still approximately valid.

4.2.3 Adaptive Design with Classifier Biomarker

4.2.3.1 Strong α-Controlled Method

Let the hypothesis test for biomarker-positive subpopulation at the first stage (size = n_1/group) be

$$H_{o1}: \delta_+ \leq 0 \tag{4.16}$$

and the hypothesis test for overall population (size = N_1/group) be

$$H_o: \delta \leq 0 \tag{4.17}$$

with the corresponding stagewise p-values, p_{1+} and p_1, respectively. These stagewise p-values should be adjusted. A conservative way is used Bonferroni method or a method similar to Dunnett method that takes the correlation into consideration. For Bonferroni-adjusted p-value and MSP, the test statistic is $T_1 = 2\min(p_{1+}, p_1)$ for the first stage. The population with a smaller p-value will be chosen for the second stage and the test statistic for the second stage is defined as $T_2 = T_1 + p_2$, where p_2 is the stagewise p-value from the second stage. This method is implemented in SAS (see Appendix).

Example 4.1 Biomarker-Adaptive Design
Suppose in an active-control trial, the estimated treatment difference is 0.2 for the BPP and 0.1 for the BNP with a common standard deviation of $\sigma = 1$. Using SAS macro in the Appendix at the end of this chapter, we can generate the operating characteristics under the global null hypothesis H_o (u0p = 0, u0n = 0), the null configurations H_{o1} (u0p = 0, u0n = 0.1) and H_{o2} (u0p = 0.2, u0n = 0), and the alternative hypothesis H_a (u0p = 0.2, u0n = 0.1) (see Table 4.2). Typical SAS macro calls to simulate the global null and the alternative conditions are presented as follows:

TABLE 4.2: Simulation results of two-stage design.

Case	FSP	ESP	Power	AveN	pPower	oPower
H_o	0.876	0.009	0.022	1678	0.011	0.011
H_{o1}	0.538	0.105	0.295	2098	0.004	0.291
H_{o2}	0.171	0.406	0.754	1852	0.674	0.080
H_a	0.064	0.615	0.908	1934	0.311	0.598

H_{o1} and H_{o2} = no effect for BPP and overall population.

»SAS»
Title "Simulation under global Ho, 2-stage design";
%BMAD(nSims=100000, CntlType="strong", nStages=2, u0p=0,
    u0n=0, sigma=1.414, np1=260, np2=260, nn1=520, nn2=520,
    alpha1=0.01, beta1=0.15, alpha2=0.1871);

Title "Simulations under Ha, 2-stage design";
%BMAD(nSims=100000, CntlType="strong", nStages=2, u0p=0.2,
    u0n=0.1, sigma=1.414, np1=260, np2=260, nn1=520, nn2=520,
    alpha1=0.01, beta1=0.15, alpha2=0.1871);
«SAS«

To generate the corresponding results for the classic single-stage design (see Table 4.3 for the simulation results), we can use the SAS calls as follows:

»SAS»
Title "Simulations under global Ho, single-stage design";
%BMAD(nSims=100000, CntlType="strong", nStages=1, u0p=0,
u0n=0, sigma=1.414, np1=400, np2=0, nn1=800, nn2=0, alpha1=0.025);

Title "Simulations under Ha, single-stage design";
%BMAD(nSims=100000, CntlType="strong", nStages=1, u0p=0.2,
u0n=0.1, sigma=1.414, np1=400, np2=0, nn1=800, nn2=0, alpha1=0.025);
«SAS«

Trial monitoring is particularly important for these types of trials. Assume that we have decided the sample sizes N_2 per treatment group for overall population

TABLE 4.3: Simulation results of classic single-stage design.

Case	FSP	ESP	Power	AveN	pPower	oPower
H_o	0.878	0.022	0.022	2400	0.011	0.011
H_{o1}	0.416	0.274	0.274	2400	0.003	0.271
H_{o2}	0.070	0.741	0.741	2400	0.684	0.056
H_a	0.015	0.904	0.904	2400	0.281	0.623

H_{o1} and H_{o2} = no effect for BPP and overall population.

at stage 2, of which n_2 (can be modified later) subjects per group are biomarker-positive. Ideally, decision on whether the trial continues for the biomarker-positive patients or overall patients should be dependent on the expected utility at the interim analysis. The utility is the total gain (usually as a function of observed treatment effect) subtracted by the cost due to continuing the trial using BPP or the overall patient population. For simplicity, we define the utility as the conditional power. The population group with larger conditional power will be used for the second stage of the trial. Suppose we design a trial with $n_{1+} = 260$, $n_{1-} = 520$, $p_{1+} = 0.1$, $p_1 = 0.12$, and stopping boundaries: $\alpha_1 = 0.01$, $\beta_1 = 0.15$, and $\alpha_2 = 0.1871$. For $n_{2+} = 260$, and $n_{2-} = 520$, the conditional power based on MSP is 82.17% for BPP and 99.39% for the overall population. The calculations are presented as follows:

$$P_c(p_1,\delta) = 1 - \Phi\left[\Phi^{-1}(1 - \alpha_2 + p_1) - \frac{\delta}{\sigma}\sqrt{\frac{n_2}{2}}\right], \quad \alpha_1 < p_1 \le \beta_1.$$

For the BPP,

$$\Phi^{-1}(1 - 0.1871 + 0.1) = \Phi^{-1}(0.9129) = 1.3588, 0.2\sqrt{260/2} = 2.2804,$$

$$P_c = 1 - \Phi(1.3588 - 2.2804) = 1 - \Phi(-0.9216) = 1 - 0.1783 = 0.8217.$$

For the BNP,

$$\Phi^{-1}(1 - 0.1871 + 0.12) = \Phi^{-1}(0.9329) = 1.4977,$$

$$0.2\sqrt{(260 + 520)/2} = 3.9497,$$

$$P_c = 1 - \Phi(1.4977 - 3.9497) = 1 - \Phi(-2.452) = 1 - 0.0071 = 0.9929.$$

Therefore, we are interested in the overall population. Of course, different n_2 and N_2 can be chosen at the interim analyses, which may lead to different decisions regarding the population for the second stage.

The following aspects should also be considered during design: power versus utility, enrolled patients versus screened patients, screening cost, and the prevalence of biomarker.

4.3 Challenges in Biomarker Validation

4.3.1 Classic Design with Biomarker Primary-Endpoint

Given the characteristics of biomarkers, can we use a biomarker as the primary endpoint for late-stage or confirmatory trials? Let us study the outcome in three different scenarios: (1) the treatment has no effect on the true endpoint or the biomarker; (2) the treatment has no effect on the true endpoint but does affect the biomarker; and

TABLE 4.4: Issues with biomarker primary endpoint.

Effect Size Ratio	Endpoint	Power (α)
0.0/0.0	True endpoint	(0.025)
	Biomarker	(0.025)
0.0/0.4	True endpoint	(0.025)
	Biomarker	(0.810)
0.2/0.4	True endpoint	0.300
	Biomarker	0.810

Note: $N = 100$ per group. Effect size ratio = effect size of true endpoint to effect size of biomarker.

(3) the treatment has a small effect on the true endpoint but has a larger effect on the biomarker. Table 4.4 summarizes the type-I error rates (α) and powers for using the true endpoint and biomarker under different scenarios. In the first scenario, we can use either the true endpoint or biomarker as the primary endpoint because both control the type-I error. In the second scenario, we cannot use the biomarker as the primary endpoint because α will be inflated to 81%. In the third scenario, it is better to use the biomarker as the primary endpoint from a power perspective. However, before the biomarker is fully validated, we do not know which scenario is true; use of the biomarker as the primary endpoint could lead to a dramatic inflation of the type-I error. It must be validated before a biomarker can be used as a primary endpoint.

4.3.2 Translation among Biomarker, Treatment, and True Endpoint

Validation of biomarker is not an easy task. Validation here refers to the proof of a biomarker to be a predictive marker, i.e., a marker can be used as a surrogate marker. Before we discuss biomarker validations, let us take a close look at the three-way relationships among treatment, biomarker, and the true endpoint. It is important to be aware that the correlations between them are not transitive. In the following example, we will show that it could be the case that there is a correlation (R_{TB}) between treatment and the biomarker and a correlation (R_{BE}) between the biomarker and the true endpoint, but there is no correlation (R_{TE}) between treatment and the true endpoint (Figures 4.1 and 4.2).

The hypothetical example to be discussed is a trial with 14 patients, 7 in the control group and 7 in the test group. The biomarker and true endpoint outcomes are displayed in Figure 4.2. The results show that Pearson's correlation between the biomarker and the true endpoint is 1 (perfect correlation) in both treatment groups. If the data are pooled from the two groups, the correlation between the biomarker and the true endpoint is still high, about 0.9. The average response with the true endpoint is 4 for each group, which indicates that the drug is ineffective when compared with the control. On the other hand, the average biomarker response is 6 for the test group and 4 for the control group, which indicates that the drug has effects on the biomarker.

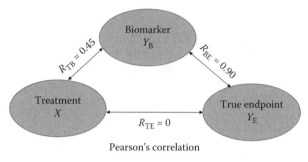

Pearson's correlation

Regression: $Y_T = Y_B - 2X$

FIGURE 4.1:   Treatment–biomarker–endpoint three-way relationship.

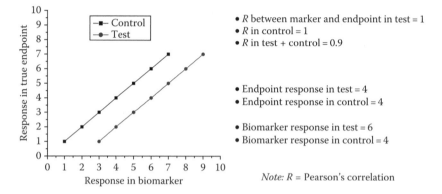

FIGURE 4.2:   Correlation versus prediction.

Facing the data, what we typically do is to fit a regression model with the data, in which the dependent variable is the true endpoint (Y_T) and the independent variables (predictors) are the biomarker (Y_B) and the treatment (X). After model fitting, we can obtain that

$$Y_T = Y_B - 2X. \tag{4.18}$$

This model fits the data well based on model-fitting p-value and R^2. Specifically, R^2 is equal to 1, p-values for model and all parameters are equal to 0, where the coefficient 2 in model (Equation 4.18) is the separation between the two lines. Based on Equation 4.18, we would conclude that both biomarker and treatment affect the true endpoint. However, we know that the treatment has no effect on biomarker at all.

In fact, the biomarker predicts the response in the true endpoint, but it does not predict the treatment effect on the true endpoint, i.e., it is a prognostic marker.

Therefore, a prognostic marker could be easily mistakenly treated as a predictive or surrogate marker. This "mis-translation" in an early clinical trial could result in a huge waste in resources for the later phase. It is also explained why there are a limit of validated surrogate makers in clinical trials.

4.3.3 Multiplicity and False-Positive Rate

Let us further discuss the challenges from a multiplicity point of view. In earlier phases or the discovery phase, we often have a large number of biomarkers to test. Running hypothesis testing on many markers can be done either with a high false-positive rate without multiplicity adjustment or a low power with multiplicity adjustment. Also, if model selection procedures are used without multiplicity adjustment as we commonly see in current practice, the false-positive rate could be inflated dramatically. Another source of false-positive discovery rate is the so-called publication bias. The last, but not the least, source of false-positive finding is due to the multiple testing conducted by different companies or research units. Imagine that 100 companies study the same biomarker; even if family-wise type-I error rate is strictly controlled at a 5% level within each company, there will still be, on average, 5 companies that have positive findings about the same biomarker just by chance.

4.3.4 Validation of Biomarkers

We have realized the importance of biomarker validation and would like to review some commonly used statistical methods for biomarker validation.

Prentice (1989) proposed four operational criteria: (1) treatment has a significant impact on the surrogate endpoint; (2) treatment has a significant impact on the true endpoint; (3) the surrogate has a significant impact on the true endpoint; and (4) the full effect of treatment on the true endpoint is captured by the surrogate endpoint. Note that this method is for a binary surrogate (Molenberghs et al., 2005).

Freedman et al. (1992) argued that the last Prentice criterion is difficult statistically because it requires that the treatment effect be not statistically significant after adjustment of the surrogate marker. They further articulated that the criterion might be useful to reject a poor surrogate marker, but it is inadequate to validate a good surrogate marker. Therefore, they proposed a different approach based on the proportion of treatment effect on true endpoint explained by biomarkers and a large proportion required for a good marker. However, as noticed by Freedman, this method is practically infeasible owing to the low precision of the estimation of the proportion explained by the surrogate.

Buyse and Molenberghs (1998) proposed the internal validation matrices, which include relative effect (RE) and adjusted association (AA). The former is a measure of association between the surrogate and the true endpoint at an individual level, and the latter expresses the relationship between the treatment effects on the surrogate and the true endpoint at a trial level. The practical use of the Buyse–Molenberghs method raises a few concerns: (1) a wide confidence interval of RE requires a large sample-size; and (2) treatment effects on the surrogate and the true endpoint are multiplicative, which cannot be checked using data from a single trial.

Other methods, such as external validation using meta-analysis and two-stage validation for fast-track programs, also face similar challenges in practice. For further readings on biomarker evaluations, Weir and Walley (2006) give an excellent review; Qu and Case (2006) proposed a method for quantifying the indirect treatment effect via surrogate markers and Alonso et al. (2006) proposed a unifying approach for surrogate marker validation based on Prentice's criteria.

There is an urgent need for a guideline from regulatory agency. To this end, several working-groups or task-force that joins efforts from industry, academia, and FDA try to develop some guidelines for biomarker qualification and validation. It is expected that in the near future, several White Paper and guideline(s) will be issued.

4.3.5 Biomarkers in Reality

In reality, there are many possible scenarios: (1) same effective size for the bio-marker and true endpoint, but the biomarker response can be measured earlier; (2) bigger effective size for the biomarker and smaller for the true endpoint; (3) no treatment effect on the true endpoint, limited treatment effect on the biomarker; and (4) treatment effect on the true endpoint only occurs after the biomarker response reaches a threshold. Validation of biomarkers is challenging, and the sample-size is often insufficient for the full validation. Therefore, validations are often performed to a certain degree and soft validation scientifically (e.g., pathway) is important.

What is the utility of partially validated biomarkers? In the next section, we will discuss how to use prognostic markers in adaptive designs.

4.4 Adaptive Design with Prognostic Biomarker

4.4.1 Optimal Design

A biomarker before it is proved predictive can only be considered as a prognostic marker. In the following example, we discuss how to use a prognostic biomarker (a marker may be predictive) in trial design. The adaptive design proposed permits early stopping for futility based on the interim analysis of the biomarker. At the final analysis, the true endpoint will be used to preserve the type-I error. Assume that there are three possible scenarios: (1) H_{o1}: effect size ratio ESR = 0/0, (2) H_{o2}: effect size ratio ESR = 0/0.25, and (3) H_a: effect size ratio ESR = 0.5/0.5, but biomarker response earlier. ESR is the ratio of effect size for true endpoint to the effect size for biomarker. We are going to compare three different designs: classic design and two adaptive designs with different stopping boundaries as shown in Table 4.5.

Based on simulation results (Table 4.5), we can see that the two adaptive designs reduce sample-size required under the null hypothesis. However, this comparison is not good enough because it does not consider the prior distribution of each scenario at the design stage.

We have noticed that there are many different scenarios with associated probabilities (prior distribution) and many possible adaptive designs with associated probabilistic outcomes (good and bad). Suppose we have also formed the utility function, the criteria for evaluating different designs. Now let us illustrate how we can use utility theory to select the best design under financial, time, and other constraints.

TABLE 4.5: Adaptive design with biomarker.

Design	Condition	Power	Expected N/Arm	Futility Boundary
Classic	H_{o1}		100	
	H_{o2}		100	
	H_a	0.94	100	
Adaptive	H_{o1}		75	
	H_{o2}		95	$\beta_1 = 0.5$
	H_a	0.94	100	
Adaptive	H_{o1}		55	
	H_{o2}		75	$\beta_1 = 0.1056$
	H_a	0.85	95	

TABLE 4.6: Prior knowledge about effect size.

Scenario	Effect Size Ratio	Prior Probability
H_{o1}	0/0	0.2
H_{o2}	0/0.25	0.2
H_a	0.5/0.5	0.6

TABLE 4.7: Expected utilities of different designs.

Design	Classic	Biomarker-Adaptive $\beta_1 = 0.5$	$\beta_1 = 0.1056$
Expected utility	419	441	411

Let us assume the prior probability for each of the scenarios mentioned earlier as shown in Table 4.6. For each scenario, we conduct computer simulations to calculate the probability of success and the expected utilities for each design. The results are summarized in Table 4.7.

Based on the expected utility, the adaptive design with the stopping boundary $\beta_1 = 0.5$ is the best. Of course, we can also generate more designs and calculate the expected utility for each design and select the best one.

4.4.2 Prognostic Biomarker in Designing Survival Trial

Insufficiently validated biomarker such as tumor RR can be used in oncology trial for interim decision-making whether to continue to enroll patients or not to reduce the cost. When the RR in the test group is lower, because of the correlation between RR and survival, it is reasonable to believe that the test drug will be unlikely to have survival benefit. However, even when the trial stopped earlier due to unfavorable results in RR, the survival benefit can still be tested. We have discussed this for a non-Hodgkin's lymphoma (NHL) trial.

4.5   Adaptive Design with Predictive Marker

If a biomarker is proved to be predictive, then we can use it to replace the true endpoint from the hypothesis test point of view. In other words, a proof of treatment effect on predictive marker is a proof of treatment effect on the true endpoint. However, the correlation between the effect sizes of treatment in the predictive (surrogate) marker and the true endpoints is desirable but unknown. This is one of the reasons that follow-up study on the true endpoint is highly desirable in the NDA accelerated approval program.

Changes in biomarker over time can be viewed as stochastic process (marker process) and have been used in the so-called threshold regression. A predictive marker process can be viewed as an external process that covariates with the parent process. It can be used in tracking the progress of the parent process if the parent process is latent or is only infrequently observed. In this way, the marker process forms a basis for predictive inference about the status of the parent process of clinical endpoint. The basic analytical framework for a marker process conceives of a bivariate stochastic process $\{X(t), Y(t)\}$ where the parent process $\{X(t)\}$ is one component process and the marker process $\{Y(t)\}$ is the other. Whitmore et al. (1998) investigated the failure inference based on a bivariate. Wiener model has also been used in this aspect, in which failure is governed by the first-hitting time of a latent degradation process. Lee et al. (2000) apply this bivariate marker model to CD4 cell counts in the context of AIDS survival. Hommel et al. (2005) studied a two-stage adaptive design with correlated data.

4.6   Summary and Discussion

We have discussed the adaptive designs with classifier, prognostic, and predictive markers. These designs can be used to improve the efficiency by identifying the right population, making decisions earlier to reduce the impact of failure, and delivering the efficacious and safer drugs to market earlier. However, full validation of a biomarker is statistically challenging, and sufficient validation tools are not available. Fortunately, adaptive designs with biomarkers can be beneficial even when the biomarkers are not fully validated. The Bayesian approach is an ideal solution for finding an optimal design, while computer simulation is a powerful tool for the utilization of biomarkers in trial design.

4.7 Appendix

This SAS macro is developed for simulating biomarker-adaptive trials with two parallel groups. The key SAS variables are defined as follows: **Alpha1** = early efficacy stopping boundary (one-sided), **beta1** = early futility stopping boundary, **Alpha2** = final efficacy stopping boundary, **u0p** = response difference in BPP, **u0n** = response in BNP, **sigma** = asymptotic standard deviation for the response difference, assuming homogeneous variance among groups. For binary response, sigma $= \sqrt{r_1(1-r_1) + r_2(1-r_2)}$; for Normal response, sigma $= \sqrt{2}\sigma$. **np1**, **np2** = sample sizes per group for the first and second stage for the BPP. **nn1**, **nn2** = sample sizes per group for the first and second stage for the BNP. **cntlType** = "strong," for the strong type-I error control and **cntlType** = "weak," for the weak type-I error control, **AveN** = average total sample-size (all arms combined), **pPower** = the probability of significance for BPP, **oPower** = the probability of significance for overall population.

```
%Macro BMAD(nSims=100000, cntlType="strong", nStages=2,
    u0p=0.2, u0n=0.1, sigma=1, np1=50, np2=50, nn1=100,
    nn2=100, alpha1=0.01, beta1=0.15, alpha2=0.1871);
Data BMAD;
 Keep FSP ESP Power AveN pPower oPower;
 seedx=1736; seedy=6214; u0p=&u0p; u0n=&u0n; np1=&np1;
    np2=&np2; nn1=&nn1; nn2=&nn2; sigma=&sigma;
    FSP=0; ESP=0; Power=0; AveN=0; pPower=0; oPower=0;
 Do isim=1 to &nSims;
    up1=Rannor(seedx)*sigma/Sqrt(np1)+u0p;
    un1=Rannor(seedy)*sigma/Sqrt(nn1)+u0n;
    uo1=(up1*np1+un1*nn1)/(np1+nn1);
    Tp1=up1*np1**0.5/sigma; To1=uo1*(np1+nn1)**0.5/sigma;
    T1=Max(Tp1,To1); p1=1-ProbNorm(T1);
    If &cntlType="strong" Then p1=2*p1; *Bonferroni;
    If p1>&beta1 Then FSP=FSP+1/&nSims;
    If p1<=&alpha1 Then Do;
       Power=Power+1/&nSims; ESP=ESP+1/&nSims;
       If Tp1>To1 Then pPower=pPower+1/&nSims;
       If Tp1<=To1 Then oPower=oPower+1/&nSims;
    End;
    AveN=AveN+2*(np1+nn1)/&nSims;
    If &nStages=2 And p1>&alpha1 And p1<=&beta1 Then Do;
       up2=Rannor(seedx)*sigma/Sqrt(np2)+u0p;
       un2=Rannor(seedy)*sigma/Sqrt(nn2)+u0n;
       uo2=(up2*np2+un2*nn2)/(np2+nn2);
       Tp2=up2*np2**0.5/sigma; To2=uo2*(np2+nn2)**0.5/sigma;
       If Tp1>To1 Then Do;
          T2=Tp2; AveN=AveN+2*np2/&nSims;
```

```
      End;
       If Tp1<=To1 Then Do;
          T2=To2; AveN=AveN+2*(np2+nn2)/&nSims;
       End;
        p2=1-ProbNorm(T2); Ts=p1+p2;
        If .<TS<=&alpha2 Then Do;
          Power=Power+1/&nSims;
          If Tp1>To1 Then pPower=pPower+1/&nSims;
          If Tp1<=To1 Then oPower=oPower+1/&nSims;
        End;
      End;
  End;
  Run;
  Proc Print Data=BMAD (obs=1); Run;
  %Mend BMAD;
```

References

Alonso, A, et al. 2006. A unifying approach for surrogate marker validation based on Prentice's criteria. *Stat. Med.*, 25:205–221.

Bretz, F. and Hothorn, L.A. 2002. Detecting dose-response using contrasts: Asymptotic power and sample-size determination for binary data. *Stat. Med.*, 21, 3325–3335.

Buyse, M. and Molenberghs, G. 1998. Criteria for the validation of surrogate endpoints in randomized experiments. *Biometrics*, 54:1014–1029.

Chang, M. 2007. *Adaptive Design Theory and Implementation Using SAS and R*. Chapman & Hall/CRC, Taylor & Francis, Boca Raton, FL.

Chow, S.C. and Chang, M. 2006. *Adaptive Design Methods in Clinical Trials*. Chapman & Hall/CRC, Taylor & Francis, Boca Raton, FL.

Conley, B.A. and Taube, S.E. 2004. Prognostic and predictive marker in cancer. *Dis. Markers*, 20, 35–43.

Crowder, M.J. 2001. Classical Competing Risks, Chapman & Hall/CRC, Boca Raton, FL.

De Gruttola, V.G., et al. 2001. Considerations in the evaluation of surrogate endpoints in clinical trials: Summary of a national institutes of health workshop. *Control. Clin. Trials*, 22:485–502.

Freedman, L.S., Graubard. B.I., and Schatzkin, A. 1992. Statistical validation of intermediate endpoints for chronic diseases. *Stat. Med.*, 11:167–178.

Hommel, G., Lindig, V., and Faldum, A. 2005. Two-stage adaptive designs with correlated test statistics. *J. Biopharm. Stat.*, 15:613–623.

Lee, M.-L.T., DeGruttola, V., and Schoenfeld, D. 2000. A model for markers and latent health status, *J. R. Stat. Soc., Ser B*, 62, 747–762.

Molenberghs, G., Buyse, M., and Burzykowski, T. 2005. The history of surrogate endpoint validation, In: *The Evaluation of Surrogate Endpoint*, Burzykowski T., Molenberghs M., and Buyse M. (Eds.). Springer, New York.

Pizzo, P.A. 2006. The Dean's Newsletter. Stanford University School of Medicine, Stanford, California.

Prentice, R.L. 1989. Surrogate endpoints in clinical trials: definitions and operational criteria. *Stat. Med.*, 8:431–440.

Qu, Y. and Case, M. 2006. Quantifying the indirect treatment effect via surrogate markers. *Stat. Med.*, 25:223–231.

Wang, S.J., Hung, H.M.J., and O'Neill, R.T. 2006. Adapting the sample-size planning of a phase III trial based on phase II data. *Pharm. Stat.*, 5:85–97.

Weir, C.J. and Walley, R.J. 2006. Statistical evaluation of biomarkers as surrogate endpoints: A literature review. *Stat. Med.*, 25:183–203.

Whitmore, G.A., Crowder, M.J., and Lawless, J.F. 1998. Failure inference from a marker process based on a bivariate Wiener model, *Lifetime Data Analysis*, 4:229–251.

Chapter 5

Targeted Clinical Trials

Jen-pei Liu

Contents

5.1   Introduction

Although a drug is approved is by the regulatory authorities to treat a certain disease or illness, owing to its effectiveness and safety, it may not be efficacious or safe for all the patients with that disease. In other words, there is a considerable variation among patients in the responses to the drug. Basically, even for the patient population with the same diagnosis, the responses to the drug can be generally classified into the following four categories:

1. Drug is efficacious for the patient without toxicity.

2. Drug is efficacious for the patient with toxicity.

3. Drug is not efficacious for the patient without toxicity.

4. Drug is not efficacious for the patient with toxicity.

These variations are the biological differences among the trial patients. Although factors such as age, gender, education or socioeconomic status, smoking habit, weight, sexual orientation, and underlying disease characteristics at the baseline may contribute to the variation among patients, one of the most important reasons is the genetic or genomic variations among the trial participants. As early as in 1990,

O'Brien and Dean (1997) found the genes that infer protection against HIV infection. In addition, a correlation between the variability in survival of the HIV-infected subjects with their genotypes was reported by Winkler et al. (1998). Excellent reviews on inheritance and drug response and on pharmacogenomics can be obtained from the works of Weinshilboum (2003) and Evans and McLeod (2003), respectively.

After completion of the Human Genome Project (HGP), the disease targets at the molecular level can be identified and must be utilized for the treatment of diseases (Simon and Maitournam, 2004; Maitournam and Simon, 2005; Casciano and Woodcock, 2006; Dalton and Friend, 2006; Varmus, 2006). On the other hand, diagnostic devices for detection of disease using state-of-the-art biotechnology, such as microarray, polymerase chain reaction (PCR), mRNA transcript profiling, etc., also became feasible. Therefore, the treatments, specific for the patients with the identified molecular targets, could be developed. It is hoped that the patients will benefit from the treatment without toxicity. Consequently, personalized medicine could become a reality. As a result, a targeted therapy is a type of treatment that uses the drugs or other means, such as monoclonal antibodies, for the identified molecular targets involved in the pathways of the disease pathogenesis. Targeted clinical trials are the trials that are employed to evaluate the efficacy and safety of the targeted therapies. Current paradigm to develop and evaluate a drug or a treatment uses a shot-gun approach that may not be beneficial for most of the patients. On the other hand, the targeted therapy employs a guided-missile approach to reach the molecular targets. As a result, for a targeted therapy or a targeted clinical trial, one must have (1) the knowledge of the involvement of the identified molecular targets in the disease pathogenesis, (2) a device for the detection of the molecular targets, and (3) a treatment developed for the molecular targets. Development of targeted therapies involves translation from the accuracy of diagnostic devices for the molecular targets to the efficacy and safety of the treatment modality for the patient population with the targets. Therefore, evaluation of targeted therapies is much more complex than that of the traditional drugs. To address the issues of development of the targeted therapies, the United States Food and Drug Administration (U.S. FDA) issued Drug-Diagnostic Co-Development Concept Paper and In Vitro Diagnostic Multivariate Index Assays in April 2005 and in July 2007, respectively. Examples of targeted clinical trials are given in the following section, and the statistical issues on the design and analysis of targeted clinical trials are provided in Section 5.3. Lastly, discussion and final remarks are presented in the final section.

5.2 Examples

Example 5.1 *Chronic Myelogenous Leukemia*

About 20% of the newly diagnosed leukemia in adults is chronic myeloid leukemia (CML). This disease consists of three distinct phases: a chronic phase with duration between 3 and 6 years, followed by an accelerated phase, and then a blast crisis during which the differentiation ability of the leukemia is lost. Allogeneic stem-cell transplantation is currently the only curable treatment for CML. However, the risk associated with allogeneic stem-cell transplantation is significant mortality and morbidity. In addition, suitable matched donors are only available for 30% of CML patients. Interferon (IFN)-α was the approved first-line therapy with only a 5%–20% complete cytogenic response rate accompanied with serious adverse events. The second-line agents, including hyroxyurea or busulfan, after the failure of IFN-α, rarely induce any cytogenic responses.

"Philadelphia (Ph+) chromosome" occurs in 90% of CML patients, which signifies a reciprocal translocation between the long arms of chromosomes 9 and 22. The direct consequence of this genetic abnormality is the formation of a *BCR-ABL* fusion gene and the generation of the fusion BCR-ABL protein. The fusion BCR-ABL protein can be found in almost all CML patients, because it is a constitutively activated tyrosine kinase with an important role in the regulation of cell growth. It has been verified by both *in vitro* studies and animal models that BCR-ABL tyrosine kinase alone is sufficient to induce CML. On the other hand, the tyrosine kinase activity is required for its oncogenic activity, as revealed by the mutational analysis. Owing to the above-mentioned possible mechanisms, the effective treatments for CML could be from the inhibitors of the BCR-ABL tyrosine kinase.

One of the selective and competitive inhibitors of the BCR-ABL protein tyrosine kinase is imatinib mesylate. From certain phase I and phase II trials, it was observed that after the failure of previous treatments of IFN-α, imatinib mesylate at 400 mg per day was capable of inducing a 60% major cytogenic response rate in the patients with confirmed late, chronic-phase CML. In addition, a 95% complete-hematologic response rate was observed in the CML patients (Druker et al., 2001; Kantarjian et al., 2002). As imatinib mesylate was the first drug that successfully treated the patients with the identified molecular targets, under the "accelerated approval" regulations for serious or life-threatening illnesses, on May 10, 2001, this drug was approved by the U.S. FDA for oral treatment of the patients with CML, based on the results of surrogate cytogenic and hematologic endpoints from the three separate single-arm studies with the database of about 1000 patients.

On the other hand, it was observed that KIT activation occurs in all the cases of gastrointestinal stromal tumors (GIST) (Rubin et al., 2001). One of the selective inhibitors of the transmembrane receptor kit is imatinib mesylate too. From a phase II study, Demetri et al. (2002) reported that 400 or 600 mg of imatinib mesylate daily can provide a 54% partial response rate in the patients with advanced GIST. Therefore, on February 1, 2002, imatinib mesylate was also approved by the U.S. FDA for the indication of the oral treatment of patients with GIST.

Despite the fact that the genetic mechanism for CML and its molecular target are quite clear, cytogenetic or hematologic responses are not observed in all the patients. Even in the case of the responders, the extent of responses and time required to reach the responses also vary. This indicates that considerable variation in responses to treatment of imatinib mesylate still exists among the patients with CML. In other words, in addition to "Philadelphia (Ph+) chromosome," *BCR-ABL* fusion gene, and its product, BCR-ABL tyrosine kinase, other causes for CML may be possible. Furthermore, after a successful induction of responses, resistance to imatinib mesylate was observed to occur in a fair amount of the patients. As a result, variation of the

BCR-ABL fusion gene and its interaction with other known or unknown genes may cause the variation in responses and resistance of the CML patients to the treatment of imatinib mesylate.

Example 5.2   *Breast Cancer*

5.2.1   Metastatic Cancer

It is estimated that in the United States, approximately 1.6 million women have been diagnosed with breast cancer. In addition, each year there are about 200,000 new cases. Furthermore, more than 40,000 women die of metastatic breast cancer each year in the United States, despite the recent advances in the diagnosis and treatment of breast cancers (Hortobagyi, 1998). Death from breast cancer accounts for about 15% of all cancer-related death in women in the United States. In most of the patients with metastatic breast cancers, objective responses can be induced by chemotherapy. However, almost all the chemotherapies are cytotoxic and can cause irreversible, serious adverse events with a high risk of death.

Human epidermal growth-factor receptor (*HER2*) is a growth-factor receptor gene that encodes the HER2 protein found on the surface of some normal cells that plays an important role in the regulation of cell growth. Furthermore, this encoded protein is present in abnormally high levels in the cancerous cells. Therefore, *HER2* is amplified in about 20%–30% of the patients with metastatic breast cancer. In addition, studies have showed that the patients with metastatic breast cancer with over-expressed *HER2* have an aggressive form of the cancer. Also, the tumors with over-expressed *HER2* are more likely to recur and the patients have statistically significant shorter progression-free survival (PFS) and overall survival (OS) (Seshadri et al., 1993; Ravdin and Chamness, 1995). Since the over-expression of *HER2* gene is a prognostic and predictive marker for the clinical outcomes, it also provides a target to search for an inhibitor for HER2 protein, as a treatment for the patients with metastatic breast cancer.

Herceptin is a recombinant DNA-derived humanized monoclonal antibody that selectively binds with high affinity to the extracellular domain of HER2 protein in a cell-based assay. To minimize immunogenecity, its anti-binding region was fused to the framework region of IgG. Both *in vitro* and *in vivo*, Herceptin was tested against breast cancer cells with over-expressed *HER2*. As a monotherapy, Herceptin was found to inhibit the tumor growth. In addition, when used in combination with other chemoagents, such as paclitaxel, it provided additive effects. Phase I studies demonstrated that the safety profile of Herceptin was tolerable. Phase II trials showed that the objective response of Herceptin was about 15% in the patients with metastatic breast cancer, after failure of the previous chemotherapy. Therefore, several large-scale, randomized phase III trials were conducted in the patients with metastatic breast cancer with over-expressed HER2 protein to confirm the effectiveness and safety of Herceptin (Slamon et al., 2001).

Enrichment design (Chow and Liu, 2004) was actually employed in these studies to compare the effects of Herceptin plus chemotherapy with chemotherapy alone.

During the enrichment phase, immunohistochemical (IHC) assay was used to screen the patients with the over-expressed *HER2*. In particular, only the patients with a weak-to-moderate staining of the entire tumor-cell membrane for *HER2* (score of 2+) or more than moderate staining (score of 3+) in more than 10% of the tumor cells on ICH analysis were randomized. The overall objective responses rates of Herceptin plus chemotherapy was 50%, which is statistically and significantly higher than the 32% observed in the patients assigned to chemotherapy alone. At one year, the OS rate was 78% for Herceptin plus chemotherapy and 67% for chemotherapy alone. Furthermore, the difference in the OS rates between the two treatments at one year was statistically significant. In addition, the patients with the highest levels of HER2 protein respond best to the treatment of Herceptin. Since congestive heart failure occurred in 27% of the patients receiving Herceptin in combination with anthracyclines and cyclophosphamide (AC), Herceptin was not approved to be used with AC by the U.S. FDA in 1998. Because the treatment of Herceptin is only designated for the patients with over-expressed HER2 protein, it is extremely critical to develop accurate, reliable, and yet inexpensive devices or assays for the detection of the over-expressed *HER2* protein, and to achieve this goal with acceptable sensitivity and specificity. Bazell (1998) described the details of ups and downs on the development of Herceptin.

As mentioned earlier, Herceptin was approved by the U.S. FDA for patients with metastatic breast cancer, associated with an over-expression of HER2 protein. However, the indication of Herceptin was expanded to the patients with early stage of breast cancer after primary therapy. The evidence of effectiveness for this patient population comes from two NCI-Cooperative Group studies (NSABP B31 and NCCTG N9831). Both the studies employed the enrichment design, which restricted enrolment of women whose breast cancer demonstrated 3+ over-expression of HER2 protein, observed either by IHC assay or gene amplification by FISH (fluorescence *in situ* hybridization). All the patients received the standard adjuvant chemotherapy that consists of four 21-day cycles of doxorubicin and AC, followed by paclitaxel administrated weekly or every 3 weeks for a total of 12 weeks. Both the studies employed a randomized, two-parallel group design, which compared the standard adjuvant chemotherapy plus Herceptin with the standard adjuvant chemotherapy alone (no treatment control). The treatment of Herceptin included Herceptin at 4 mg/kg on the day of paclitaxel initiation and subsequently at 2 mg/kg for a total of 52 weeks.

The primary endpoint was the disease-free survival (DFS), which is defined as the time from randomization to recurrence, occurrence of contralateral breast cancer, other second primary cancer, or death. The total number of primary endpoint events for both the studies combined was 710, which can provide a 90% power to detect a 25% reduction in the event rate. The first combined interim analysis was scheduled after the accumulation of half of the prespecified total number of events. Subsequent combined interim analyses were scheduled every 6 months. The nominal *p*-value corresponding to the boundary for early termination for superior efficacy was 0.0001. In April 2005, the Data Monitoring Committee recommended that the results of the combined interim analysis be made public, because of superior efficacy observed in the arm of Herceptin plus standard-adjuvant chemotherapy.

For the combined studies, there were a total of 3351 patients, where 1672 and 1679 patients were randomized to Herceptin plus standard adjuvant chemotherapy or standard adjuvant chemotherapy alone, respectively. The number of primary endpoint events was 133 in the group receiving Herceptin plus standard adjuvant chemotherapy and was 261 for the standard adjuvant chemotherapy. The estimated hazard ratio was 0.48 with a corresponding 95% confidence interval from 0.39 to 0.59. The *p*-value for the reduction of the hazard ratio was <0.0001, which is smaller than that for early termination (Romond et al., 2005). In addition, 62 deaths occurred in the group of Herceptin plus the standard adjuvant chemotherapy and the number of deaths for the group receiving standard adjuvant chemotherapy was 92. The hazard ratio of death was 0.67 with a corresponding 95% confidence interval from 0.48 to 0.93 and a *p*-value of 0.015. The OS rate at 4 years was 91.4% for the group of Herceptin plus the standard adjuvant chemotherapy and was 86.6% for the group receiving only the standard adjuvant chemotherapy. Owing to its significant prolongation in DFS, the U.S. FDA, on November 16, 2006, approved Herceptin to be used as a part of the treatment of regimen containing doxorubicin, AC, and paclitaxel for the adjuvant treatment of women with node-positive, *HER2*-over-expressing breast cancer.

5.2.2   ALTTO Trial

Although Herceptin is efficacious for the patients with over-expression of *HER2* gene, some patients still do not respond or developed resistance to the treatment of Herceptin. However, Lapatinib is a second-generation drug, which is designed for multiple targets. It is a small molecule and a tyrosine kinase inhibitor that binds to part of the *HER2* protein beneath the surface of the cancer cell. It may have the ability to cross the blood–brain barrier to inhibit the spread of breast cancer to the brain and central nervous system that Herceptin fails to do. In March 2007, lapatinib was approved by the U.S. FDA in combination with capecitabine for the patients with advanced or metastatic breast cancer and over-expression of *HER2* gene, who have received prior treatment.

As mentioned earlier, *HER2*-positive tumors affect about 20%–25% patients with breast cancer. Currently, there are two agents approved to treat the patients of breast cancer with over-expression of *HER2* gene. However, the questions on which agent is more effective, which drug is safer, whether additional benefits can be obtained if two agents are administrated together, and in what order still remain unanswered. To address these issues, the U.S. National Cancer Institute and the Breast International Group (BIG) launch a new study dubbed ALTTO (Adjuvant Lapatinib and/or Trastuzumab Treatment Optimization) trial. This is a randomized, open-label, active control, and parallel study conducted in 1300 centers of 50 countries with a pre-planned enrolment of 8000 patients (ALTTO trial, 2008a–c). This study has two different patient populations depending on whether their stage I or stage II breast cancer has already been treated with chemotherapy. The patients enrolled in the ALTTO study would receive study treatment for 52 weeks with a follow-up period of 10 years.

The following criteria are employed by the central laboratory to identify the over-expression and/or amplification of *HER2* gene in the invasive component of the primary tumor, prior to randomization:

1. 3+ over-expression by IHC (>30% of invasive tumor cells), or

2. 2+ or 3+ (in ≤ 30% neoplastic cells) over-expression by IHC and FISH test demonstrating *HER2* gene amplification, or

3. *HER2* gene amplification by FISH (>6 *HER2* gene copies per nucleus or a FISH ratio of >2.2).

The primary endpoint of the ALTTO study is the DFS and the secondary endpoints include OS, serious or sever adverse events, cardiovascular events, such as heart attacks or strokes, and incidence of brain metastasis. The four treatments are

1. Standard treatment of Herceptin for 1 year

2. Lapatinib alone for 1 year

3. Herceptin for 12 weeks followed by a washout period of 6 weeks and then lapatinib for 34 weeks

4. Herceptin and Lapatinib together for 1 year

However, some patients in all groups would receive paclitaxel every week for 3 months. Hormonal therapy is at the discretion of the treating physician and would be started after the patient completes the treatment of paclitaxel and would continue for at least 5 years.

As stated in the NIH press release on February 29, 2008, the ALTTO trial is one of the first trials with a scope, in which translation research plays a critical role. In addition, the biological samples collected from the patients enrolled in the ALTTO trial will determine a tumor profile that responds best to the drugs. This vital information could lead to individualized treatment of the patients and possibly to the development of next generation drugs.

5.2.3 TAILORx Trial

Currently, the absolute expression levels of estrogen receptor (ER), those of the progesterone receptor (PR, an indicator of ER pathway), and the involvement of lymph nodes are reliable predictors for the clinical outcomes of the patients with breast cancer. Over a half of newly diagnosed patients will have ER positive, lymph node negative breast cancer. Surgical incision of the tumor, followed by radiation and hormonal therapy, is the current standard treatment practice for 80%–85% of these patients. Chemotherapy is also recommended for most of these patients. However, only a very small proportion of these patients actually benefit from the toxic chemotherapy. On the other hand, currently, no accurate method exists for predicting whether chemotherapy is necessary or not for individual patients. As a result, the ability to accurately predict the outcome of chemotherapy for an individual patient should significantly advance the management of this group of patients and to achieve the goal of personalized medicine.

Oncotype DX is a reverse-transcriptase-PCR (RT-PCR) assay, which measures the levels of expression of 21 genes. These 21 genes include those involved in tumor proliferation and hormonal response. This assay can more precisely estimate the risk of recurrence of tumors than the standard characteristics, such as tumor size and grade (Paik et al., 2004). Oncotype DX transforms the levels of expression of 21 genes into a recurrence score (RS). The range of the RS is from 0 to 100, the higher the score, the higher the risk of recurrence of tumors in the patients receiving hormonal therapy. In a retrospective analysis, Paik et al. (2006) reported that for the patients with RS >31 receiving chemotherapy and hormonal treatment of tamoxifen, the relative risk (RR) of recurrence is 0.26 with the corresponding 95% confidence interval from 0.13 to 0.53 and a p-value <0.001. Therefore, adjuvant chemotherapy is beneficial for the patients with a high RS. However, the RR is 1.31 for the patients with RS <18 (p-value = 0.61). As a result, in addition to hormonal therapy, adjuvant chemotherapy is unlikely to provide any benefit to the patients with a low risk of recurrence. For the patients with RS between 19 and 30, the benefit of adjuvant chemotherapy is uncertain.

Based on the encouraging results provided by Paik et al. (2006), on May 23, 2006, the U.S. National Cancer Institute (NCI) launched the TAILORx (Trial Assigning Individualized Options for Treatment (Rx)) trial to investigate whether genes that are frequently associated with risk of recurrence in the patients with early-stage breast cancer can be employed to assign the most appropriate and effective treatment (Spranano et al., 2006). The TAILORx trial intends to enroll abound 10,000 patients with early-stage breast cancer. Based on their RS, the patients are classified into three groups with different treatments:

1. Patients with RS >25 will receive chemotherapy plus hormonal therapy.

2. Patients with RS <11 will be given hormonal therapy alone.

3. Patients with RS between 11 and 25 inclusively will be randomly assigned to hormonal therapy alone or to chemotherapy plus hormonal therapy.

The primary objectives of the TAILORx trial are

1. To compare the DFS of the patients with previously resected axillary-node-negative breast cancer with RS of 11–25, treated with adjuvant-combination chemotherapy and hormonal therapy versus adjuvant therapy alone

2. To compare the distant-free interval, recurrence-free interval, and OS of patients with RS of 11–25, treated with these regimens

3. To create a tissue and specimen bank that includes formalin-fixed, paraffin-embedded tumor specimens, tissue microarray, plasma, and DNA obtained from the peripheral blood of patients enrolled in the TAILORx trial

The major inclusion criteria include

1. Histologically confirmed adenocarcinoma of the breast

3. Estrogen and/or progesterone receptor-positive tumor

4. HER2 negative tumor, determined by either FISH or IHC (e.g., 0 or +1 by DAKO HercepTest)

5. Having undergone surgery to remove the primary tumor by either a modified radical mastectomy or local excision along with an acceptable axillary procedure

6. Tumor size of 1.1–5.0 cm

7. Tissue specimen for the primary tumor available for diagnostic testing with Oncotype DX to determine the RS

Hormonal therapy includes oral tamoxifen alone, oral aromatase inhibitor (e.g., anastrozole, letrozole, or exemestane) alone, or oral tamoxifen followed by oral aromatase alone, administered at the discretion of the treating physician for 5–10 years. On the other hand, the standard adjuvant-combination chemotherapy includes either taxane containing (i.e., paclitaxel or docetaxel) or non-taxane containing regiments administered at the discretion of the treating physician. For patients with RS between 11 and 25 and assigned to chemotherapy plus hormonal therapy, the hormonal therapy begins within 4 weeks of the last dose of the chemotherapy, subjected to the discretion of the treating physician.

The primary outcomes of the TAILORx trial consists of

1. DFS

2. Distant recurrence-free survival

3. Recurrence-free survival

4. OS

In summary, the TAILORx is a prospective trial, which investigates the utility of the incorporation of a molecular profiling set Oncotype DX into clinical decision-making to avoid unnecessary chemotherapy from which patients are unlikely to be benefitted. The TAILORx trial will enroll more than 10,000 patients at 900 sites in the United States. It is estimated that 44% of them will have RS between 11 and 25. The duration of treatment is 10 years with an additional follow-up of 20 years after initial therapy.

5.2.4 MINDACT Trial

The MINDACT trial stands for Microarray In Node negative Disease may Avoid ChemoTherapy trial. Sponsored by the European Organization for Research and Treatment of Cancer (EORTC), it is a prospective, randomized study comparing the 70-gene expression signature with common clinical–pathological criteria in selecting adjuvant chemotherapy in node-negative breast cancer (The MINDACT Trial, 2008). Currently, the decision for prescribing adjuvant chemotherapy for the patients with node-negative breast cancer is determined by the clinical and pathological criteria, such as tumor grade, stage, or hormone-receptor expression. Recently, new molecular markers, such as *HER2*, vascular invasion of the primary tumor, and expression levels of hormone receptor are available and incorporated into the decision-making process of determining the best treatment for the patients. However, considerable debates and disagreement exists on the importance of individual molecular markers or their clinical relevance. On the other hand, the death rate from metastatic breast cancer is almost 100%. As a result, current guidance intends to avoid undertreatment of the patients with breast cancer. This results in possible overtreatment and diminishing quality of life for many patients with breast cancer and at the same time increases the avoidable disease burden on society.

The MINDACT trial employs a device, MammaPrint, which is a qualitative *in vitro* diagnostic test using the expression profile of 70 genes from fresh, frozen breast-cancer tissue samples, based on microarray technology to assess the risk of distant metastasis in patients with node-negative breast cancer (Van de Vijver et al., 2002; van't Veer et al., 2002; Buyse et al., 2006). The MammaPrint was approved by the U.S. FDA on February 2007 as a Class II device. Based on the sample expression profile, the MammaPrint computes the MammaPrint index, which is a correlation of sample profile with the "Low Risk" template profile. The MammaPrint index has a range from -1 to $+1$. Tumor samples with a MammaPrint index $\leq +0.4$ are classified as high risk for distant metastasis. Otherwise, the tumor samples are classified as low risk.

Eligibility criteria for the MINDACT trial include the following:

1. Women with cytologically or histologically proven operable, invasive breast cancer, who have a negative sentinel node or a negative axillary clearance

2. Tumor T1, T2, or operable T3

3. Breast cancer must be unilateral

4. Authorized surgery options include

    a. Breast conserving surgery

    b. Mastectomy combined with either a sentinel node procedure or full axillary clearance

5. Availability of a frozen tumor-tissue sample (not fixation in formalin)

6. Age between 18 and 70 years

7. WHO performance status 0 or 1

8. No previous chemotherapy or radiotherapy

After meeting the eligibility criteria listed above, the patients will be assessed for their risk of distant metastasis by either

1. Clinical–pathological evaluation or

2. The 70-gene signature by MammaPrint.

If both clinical–pathological evaluation and the 70-gene signature predict a high risk of distant metastasis, then this group of patients will be included in the component of "chemotherapy randomization" of the trial. On the other hand, if both clinical–pathological evaluation and the 70-gene signature predict that the risk of distant metastasis is low, then this group of patients will be included in the component of "endocrine therapy randomization" of the study. However, patients with discordant results on the risk of distant metastasis between clinical–pathological evaluation and the 70-gene signature will be included in the component of "treatment decision randomization" of the study, which will answer the primary objective of the MINDACT trial. The patients with discordant results on the risk of distant metastasis provided by the clinical–pathological evaluation and the 70-gene signature will be randomized to a test or a control group. For the test group, the results on the risk of distant metastasis, based on the 70-gene signature from MammaPrint will be employed to determine whether the patients must receive the adjuvant chemotherapy or less-aggressive endocrine therapy. On the other hand, for the control group, the traditional clinical–pathological evaluation will be used to select the treatments, either chemotherapy or endocrine therapy, for the patients with discordant results. It is estimated that 32% of the patients will have discordant results and 10%–15% of the patients will spare the unnecessary chemotherapy.

One of the main interests in the component of "randomization-treatment decision" is focused on the group of patients who have a low risk of distant metastasis predicted by the 70-gene signature and a high risk of distant metastasis by clinical–pathological criteria, and who are randomized to use the 70-gene signature with a decision of receiving no chemotherapy. The primary endpoint for this portion of the trial is distant metastasis free survival (DMFS). The null hypothesis is that the 5-year DMFS is 92%. With an accrual of 3 years and a total duration of 6 years, a sample size of 672 patients will provide an 80% power to detect an improvement of the 5-year DMFS to 95% for a one-sided test at the 2.5% significance level.

The primary objective of the component "chemotherapy randomization" in the MINDACT trial is to compare a docetaxel-capecitabine regimen with the anthracycline-based chemotherapy regimens. The primary endpoint for this component is PFS. Based on the assumption that the 5-year DFS of anthracycline-based chemotherapy regimens is 86%, a total sample size of 4000 patients will provide an 80% power to detect a hazard ratio of 0.86 (or 89% of the docetaxel-capecitabine regimen) for a two-sided test at the 5% significance level.

The primary objective of the component "endocrine therapy randomization" in the MINDACT trial is to compare regimens of 7-year single agent of Letrozole to a sequential regimen of 2 years of Tamoxifen, followed by 5 years of Letrozole. The primary endpoint for this component is PFS. Based on the assumption that the 5-year DFS of the sequential regimen of Tamoxifen followed by Letrozole is 86%, a total sample size of 3500 patients will provide an 80% power to detect a hazard ratio of 0.75 (or 89.3% of the single agent of Letrozole) for a two-sided test at the 5% significance level.

The MINDACT trial is an example of translation research for which one of the major objectives is to validate the previously discovered gene-expression profiles and a possible identification of new novel signatures. In addition, as the tissue, serum, and RNA will be collected from 6000 patients enrolled in the MINDACT trial, this provides a unique opportunity to study the gene-expression profiles for the patients either receiving the anthracycline-based chemotherapy or docetaxel-capecitabine. Therefore, it is possible, prospectively, to correlate the gene-expression profiles of these patients with the success or failure of the adjuvant-chemotherapy regimen they received. Similarly, the correlation between the gene-expression profiles and clinical outcome can be also established for the patients enrolled in the components of "endocrine therapy randomization."

Example 5.3 *Non-Small-Cell Lung Cancer*

The leading type of cancer in the world is the lung cancer. For example, approximately 173,000 persons are diagnosed with lung cancer each year in the United States. In 2005, it is estimated that 163,510 people died from lung cancer, which accounts for about 29% of all the cancer-related deaths in the United States. Therefore, lung cancer is also the leading cause of cancer-related deaths in the United States. In particular, as reported by Kris et al. (2003), more than 60,000 persons developed stage IIIB and IV non-small-cell lung cancer (NSCLC) in the United States. For patients with NSCLC receiving the best supporting care after one or more prior chemotherapy regimen, the median survival was just 16 weeks with a dismal 1-year survival rate of about 16% only (Fukuoka et al., 2003). Therefore, almost all of them will die from metastasis of the cancer. Consequently, more people die from NSCLC than those from breast, colorectal, and prostate cancer combined together.

The epidermal growth factor receptor (EGFR) is over-expressed in the cells of certain types of human tumors, including NSCLC. EGFR family of genes encodes over-expressed transmembrane molecules that may induce inappropriate activation of the anti-apoptotic RAS signal-transduction cascade and consequently lead to uncontrollable cell proliferation. Patients suffering from NSCLC with an over-expression of EGFR gene usually have very poor clinical outcomes. For this reason, it is of clinical interest and significance to search for the potent and selective inhibitors of tyrosine kinase of the EGFR.

Gefitinib is the first selective inhibitor of EGFR tyrosine kinase. Based on its promising efficacious results and tolerable safety profiles from phase II trials, it was approved by the U.S. FDA on May 5, 2003 under the accelerated approval (Subpart H) program for the treatment of patients with NSCLC, who had failed one or more courses of chemotherapy. One of the requirements for the FDA accelerated approval of gefitinib was that the sponsor must investigate the drug further after approval to verify the expected clinical benefit. As a result, the sponsor of gefitinib conducted a study in approximately 1700 patients to determine whether gefitinib would in fact prolong the survival in comparison with the patients receiving placebo. On December 17, 2004, the sponsor announced the initial analysis of the primary endpoint of Study 709, IRESSA Survival Evaluation in Lung cancer (ISEL). With 1692 patients, the results showed that the median survival time of gefitinib was 5.6 months when compared with 5.1 months for the placebo group. As a result, the hazard ratio of survival of gefitinib compared with the placebo was 0.89 with a p-value of 0.11. Thus, Study 709 failed to provide evidence to support that gefitinib can prolong the survival of the patients with NSCLC. The results of the Iressa NSCLC Trial Assessing Combination Treatment (INTACT) 2 also failed to support that gefitinib in combination with paclitaxel and carboplatin provides added clinical benefit in OS, time-to-progression, and response rate in the chemotherapy-naïve patients with advanced NSCLC (Herbst et al., 2004). Because of the failure to extend the survival for majority of the patients with NSCLS, on June 17, 2005 the U.S. FDA revised the labeling of gefitinib, restricting the administration to cancer patients who, in the opinion of their physician, are currently benefiting, or have previously benefited, from gefitinib treatment.

Erlotinib is another selective and potent inhibitor that targets the EGFR pathway. The National Cancer Institute of Canada Trials Group (NCI CTG) conducted an international, phase III, randomized, double-blind, placebo-controlled study (BR.21) to investigate the efficacy of erlotinib in the patients with NSCLC after failure of first-line or second-line chemotherapy. The primary endpoint is OS and secondary endpoints include PFS, overall response rate, duration of response, safety profiles, and quality of life. Patients were randomized in a 2:1 ratio to receive either erlotinib or placebo. A total sample size of 700 patients with expected total number of deaths of 582 would provide 90% power to detect a 33% improvement in the median survival for a two-sided test at the 5% significance level. A total of 731 patients were randomized, with 488 receiving erlotinib and 243 receiving placebo. In addition, a total of 328 patients were tested for expression of EGFR, which was determined by means of IHC assay. A tumor is considered positive for EGFR if $>10\%$ of tumor cells showed membranous staining of any intensity (Shepherd et al., 2005).

The results of Study BR.21 showed that the median OS of the patients receiving erlotinib was 5.7 months and was 4.7 months for the placebo group (Shepherd et al., 2005). The hazard ratio of death of erlotinib group was 0.70 with a p-value <0.001 and a 95% confidence interval from 0.58 to 0.85. The hazard ratio of PFS of erlotinib group was 0.61 with a p-value <0.001 and a 95% confidence interval from 0.51 to 0.74. The overall response rate was 8.9% for the erlotinib group and $<1\%$ for the placebo group with a p-value <0.001. In addition, the results of Study BR.31 indicated that superior efficacy of erlotinib is associated with females, nonsmokers, Asian origin, and patients with adenocarcinoma (Shepherd et al., 2005). In addition, Tsao et al. (2005) determined that the clinical benefit as measured by OS is correlated significantly with the EGFR positivity and amplification of EGFR. Therefore, the expression level and number of copies of EGFR may serve as the potential markers for the clinical benefits in the patients receiving treatment with erlotinib.

5.3   Statistical Considerations

5.3.1   Accuracy of Diagnostic Devices for Molecular Targets

For the traditional clinical trials, inclusion and exclusion criteria are usually based on some clinical endpoints, such as level of fasting plasma glucose or diastolic blood pressure to define the patient population in which the new treatments are evaluated, against the concurrent controls. However, as illustrated by examples given earlier, the clinical signs, symptoms, or other endpoints, such as tumor grades, positive lymph nodes, and metastasis for breast cancer, are not sufficiently correlated with the clinical benefits of the treatments in the patient population defined by the clinical-based inclusion and exclusion criteria. One of the many possible reasons is that the variability of the patient population defined by the traditional clinical endpoints is so huge that most of the patients will not benefit from the treatment, but at the same time are at a greater risk of some serious adverse effects. In other words, some patients in the patient population, defined by traditional clinical endpoints, are not suited for this treatment.

Recent advances and breakthroughs in the biomedical science and biotechnology lead us to understand the mechanisms of the disease pathways and identify the molecular targets of the disease. As a result, assays for identification of molecular targets are included as inclusion or exclusion criteria of the clinical trials to define the patient population. For example, IHC assay or FISH are used for identification of the patients who suffer from breast cancer with over-expression of HER2 protein in the study NSABP B31 and NCCTG N9831. On the other hand, the TAILORx used the RS obtained from Oncotype DX, an RT-PCR assay, to measure the expression level of 21 genes to classify patients with early-stage breast cancer into three groups with different risk of recurrence; and the MINDACT study employed the MammaPrint Index from the MammaPrint to identify the risk of distant metastasis for early-stage breast cancer. Although understanding and identification of molecular targets allow us to more precisely define the patient population than the traditional clinical endpoints, the same issue still remains unanswered. This is because no diagnostic test or assays is 100% accurate and the gold standard for diagnosis of the molecular targets is not yet established.

Table 5.1 provides the concordant results on detection of over-expression of *HER2* gene by clinical trial assay (CTA), DAKO HercepTest (P980018), InSite[TM] Her-2/neu (P040030), and PathVysion Kit (P980024/S001). The CTA was an investigational IHC assay used in the Herceptin clinical trials. The CTA uses a four-point ordinal score system (0, 1+, 2+, 3+) to measure the intensity of the expression of *HER2* gene. A score of 2+ is assigned to the weak-to-moderate staining of the entire tumor-cell membrane for HER2 in >10% of tumor cells. Patients with moderate staining in >10% of tumor cells have a CTA score of 3+. Only the patients with a CTA score of 2+ or 3+ were eligible for the Herceptin clinical trials (Slamon et al., 2001). Both DAKO HercepTest and InSite Her-2/neu are IHC assay with the same four-point ordinal score system as the CTA. On the other hand, PathVysion Kit is a FISH assay with a binary outcome (− or +). Because the results of these

TABLE 5.1: Concordant results in detection of HER2 gene.

Comparison: DAKO HercepTest versus Clinical Trial Assay

HercerpTest	Clinical Trial Assay			Total
	≤1	2	3	
≤1	215 (39.2%)	50 (9.1%)	8 (1.5%)	273 (49.8%)
2	53 (9.7%)	57 (10.4%)	16 (2.9%)	126 (23.0%)
3	6 (1.1%)	36 (6.6%)	107 (19.5%)	149 (27.2%)
Total	274 (50.0%)	143 (26.1%)	131 (23.9%)	548

Comparison: InSite Her-2/neu versus DAKO HercepTest

InSite Her-2/neu	HercerpTest			Total
	≤1	2	3	
≤1	128 (39.2%)	5 (1.4%)	2 (0.6%)	135 (38.4%)
2	25 (7.1%)	80 (22.7%)	9 (2.6%)	114 (32.4%)
3	11 (3.1%)	14 (4.0%)	78 (22.2%)	103 (29.2%)
Total	274 (46.6%)	99 (28.1%)	89 (25.3%)	352

Comparison: PathVysion Kit (FISH) versus Clinical Trial Assay

FISH	Clinical Trial Assay			Total
	≤1	2	3	
−	235 (44.4%)	67 (12.7%)	21 (4.0%)	323 (61.1%)
+	9 (1.7%)	21 (4.0%)	176 (33.3%)	206 (38.9%)
Total	244 (46.1%)	88 (16.7%)	197 (32.3%)	529

Source: From FDA Decision Summary P980018, Rockville, Maryland, 1998; FDA Decision Summary P980024/S001, Rockville, Maryland, 2001; FDA Decision Summary P040030, Rockville, Maryland, 2004.

assays have significant impact on the clinical outcomes, such as death or serious adverse events, they are classified as Class III devices, which require clinical trials as mandated by the premarket approval (PMA) of the U.S. FDA. From Table 5.1, considerable inconsistency in identification of over-expression of *HER2* gene exists among the three assays. For example, if a cutoff of ≥2+ is used for the detection of over-expression of *HER2* gene, then a total of 21.4% (117/548) of the samples would have discordant results between CTA and DAKO HercepTest. In other words, owing to the different results in the detection of over-expression of *HER2* gene, an incorrect decision for selection of treatments will be made for at least one out of five patients with metastasis breast cancer. Even if a more stringent threshold of 3+ is used, discordant results would still occur in 12.1% of the samples. Similar observations of inconsistence can be found between HercepTest and InSite™ Her-2/neu.

For comparison of the results between the two technology platforms, i.e., the CTA versus PathVysion Kit, if a score of ≥2+ is used as the cutoff, discordant results

TABLE 5.2:   Treatment effects as a function of HER2 over-expression or amplification.

HER2 Assay Result	Number of Patients	RR for Mortality (95% CI)
CTA 2+ or 3+	469	0.80 (0.64, 1.00)
FISH(+)	325	0.70 (0.53, 0.91)
FISH(−)	126	1.06 (0.70, 1.63)
CTA 2+	120	1.26 (0.82, 1.94)
FISH(+)	32	1.31 (0.53, 3.27)
FISH(−)	126	1.11 (0.68, 1.82)
CTA 3+	329	0.70 (0.51, 0.90)
FISH(+)	293	0.67 (0.51, 0.89)
FISH(−)	43	0.88 (0.39, 1.98)

Source: From FDA Annotated Redlined Draft Package Insert for Herceptin, Rockville, Maryland, 2006.

would occur in 16.7% of the patients. On the other hand, 9.7% of the patients will have inconsistent results for identification of over-expression of *HER2* gene between the CTA and PathVysion Kit, if a threshold of 3+ is employed for the CTA.

Table 5.2 provides a summary of the RR of mortality between the Herceptin plus chemotherapy group and the chemotherapy group, as a function of *HER2* over-expression by the CTA assay or amplification by FISH from Study 3 in one of the Herceptin clinical trials provided in the U.S. Package Insert of Herceptin (FDA, 2006). For the 293 patients with a CTA score of 3+ or a positive result by FISH, the RR for mortality is 0.67 with the corresponding 95% confidence interval from 0.51 to 0.90. Therefore, Herceptin plus chemotherapy provides a superior clinical benefit in terms of survival over mere chemotherapy alone, in this group of patients. On the other hand, for the patients with a CTA score of 2+, the RR for mortality is 1.31 and 1.11 for the patients with positive and negative FISH results, respectively. The corresponding 95% confidence intervals contain 1. These results imply that Herceptin plus chemotherapy may not provide additional survival benefit for the patients with a CTA score of 2+.

As mentioned earlier, the patients with a CTA score >2+ were eligible for Study 3. However, the results from Study 3 indicate that the Herceptin plus chemotherapy is not effective in the patients with a CTA score of 2+, irrespective of their amplification status of *HER2* gene by FISH. On the other hand, as shown in Table 5.1, there could be up to 22% of discordant results between the different assays for detection of over-expression of *HER2* gene. In addition, from the Decision Summary of HercepTest (P980018), the findings of inter-laboratory reproducibility study showed that 12 of 120 samples (10%) had discrepancy results between 2+ and 3+ staining intensity. It can be observed that some patients tested with a score of 3+ may actually have a score of 2+, and the patients tested with a score of 2+ may in fact have a score of 3+. As a result, the patient population defined by these assays is not exactly the same as those actually defined with the molecular targets, who will be benefitted from the treatments. As a result, because the patients with a CTA score 3+ may in fact have a score of 2+, the treatment effect of the Herceptin plus chemotherapy in terms of RR for mortality given in Table 5.2 might be underestimated for the patients truly with over-expression of *HER2* gene. On the other hand, the treatment effect of the Herceptin plus chemotherapy in terms of RR for mortality given in Table 5.2 might be over-estimated for the patients with a CTA score of 2+, because some of them may in fact have a CTA of score of 3+. Safety is another important issue for inaccuracy of the assay. The patients tested with a CTA score of 3+, in fact may have a CTA score of 2+ and would not only fail to benefit from the treatment of Herceptin but also are exposed to some very serious or even fatal adverse events, such as left ventricular dysfunction, congestive heart failure, dyspnea, clinical significant hypotension, anaphylaxis, pneumonitis, or acute respiratory distress syndrome.

As mentioned earlier, the MammaPrint is a Class II device which uses the gene-expression profile of the patients with breast cancer to assess a patient's risk of distant metastasis. The MammaPrint was approved in February 2007 by the U.S. FDA. One of the effectiveness evidence presented in the Decision Summary of the MammaPrint is the result of clinical sensitivity and specificity from the TRANSBIG study (Buyse et al., 2004; FDA, 2007). The positive predicted value (PPV) is computed based on the data of the TRANSBIG study. Here, the PPV is the probability that the metastatic disease would occur within a particular time frame given the device output for that patient is high risk. On the other hand, the negative predictive value (NPV) for the TRANSBIG trial is defined as the probability that the metastatic disease would not occur within a particular time frame given the device output for that patient is low risk. For the metastatic disease at 10 years, the TRANSBIG trial provides an estimate of 0.29 for the PPV with a 95% confidence interval from 0.22 to 0.35, and 0.90 for the NPV with a 95% confidence interval from 0.85 to 0.96. In other words, the patients tested positive for high risk using MammaPrint, in fact have a 71% probability that the metastatic disease would not occur within 10 years, and may receive unnecessary chemotherapy from which these patients will not be benefitted. Therefore, a futile result from the component of chemotherapy randomization of the MINDACT trial does not mean that the chemotherapy is not effective for the patients actually with high risk of metastasis. This is because 71% of the patients tested positive for high risk of distant metastasis by the MammaPrint in fact may not be at high risk at all, while the treatment effect of the chemotherapy might be underestimated for patients actually at high risk of distant metastasis.

5.3.2   Statistical Designs

From the examples given in Section 5.2, in general, there are three classes of targeted clinical trials. The first type is to evaluate the efficacy and safety of the targeted treatment for the patients with molecular targets. Herceptin clinical trials belong to this class. The second type of targeted clinical trials is to select the best treatment regimen for the patients based on the results of some tests for prognosis of clinical outcomes. The TAILORx trial and MINDACT trial can be classified into this class of the trials. The last type of the targeted clinical trials is to investigate the correlation of the treatment effect with variations of the molecular targets. The clinical

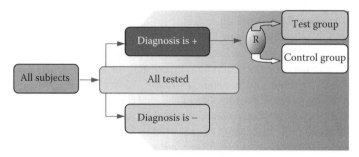

FIGURE 5.1:   Design A for targeted clinical trials.

trials given in Example 5.3 to investigate the association of the treatment effect of erlotinib as measured by the hazard ratio with the expression level and number of copies of EGFR gene are fitted into the last class. Since the objectives of different targeted clinical trials are different, the U.S. FDA Drug-Diagnostic Co-Development Concept Paper (2005) proposed three different designs to meet the different objectives of targeted clinical trials. These three designs are given in Figures 5.1 through 5.3.

Design A is the enrichment design (Chow and Liu, 2004), in which only the patients who tested positive for identification of molecular targets are randomized either to receive the test drug or the concurrent control. The enrichment design is usually employed when there is a high degree of certainty that the drug response occurs only in the patients tested positive for the molecular targets, and when the mechanism of pathological pathways is clearly understood. Most of the Herceptin phase III clinical trials used the enrichment design. However, as pointed out in the U.S. FDA Concept Paper, the description of test sensitivity and specificity will not be possible using this type of design without drug and placebo data in the patients tested negative for the molecular targets.

Design B is a stratified randomized design and stratification factor is the result of the test for the molecular targets. In other words, the patients are stratified into two groups depending on whether the diagnostic test is either positive or negative. Then, a separate randomization is independently performed within each group to

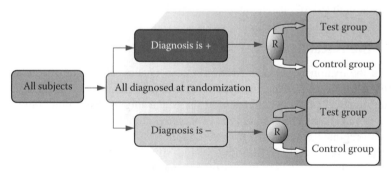

FIGURE 5.2:   Design B for targeted clinical trials.

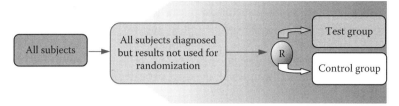

FIGURE 5.3: Design C for targeted clinical trials.

receive the test drug or concurrent control. The designs of both the TAILORx and MINDACT trials are variations of Design B. For example, in the TAILORx trial, the patients are stratified into three groups: RS <11, 11–25 inclusively, and >25. In addition, the treatments assigned to the patients are also different in these three groups. A similar design is used for the MINDACT trials, depending on the results of risk assessment for distant metastasis from clinical–pathological criteria and 70-gene signature; patients are stratified into components of treatment decision randomization, chemotherapy randomization, and endocrine therapy randomization. Within each of the components, patients are randomized to receive different treatments, while the treatments evaluated within each component are different as well.

The information of the test results for the molecular targets in Design C is primarily used as covariates and is not involved with randomization. Sometimes, only a fraction of the patients are tested for the molecular targets. Design C is useful when the association of the treatment effect of the drug with the results of the diagnostic test needs to be further explored. Study BR.21 for evaluation of erlotinib in the patients with advanced NSCLC used Design C to explore the patterns of association between the treatment effects of erlotinib, in terms of hazard ratio and amplification or expression intensity of EGFR gene.

As mentioned in the U.S. FDA concept paper, design considerations for the targeted clinical trials for the drug-device co-development should include

1. The utility of the diagnostic test, which is the strength of the association between the test results and a particular treatment response, either beneficial or toxic. The utility of the diagnostic test should be examined by the size of the difference of the treatment response between the tested and untested groups.

2. Whether patients are readily identifiable in a clinical practice setting.

3. The prevalence of the molecular targets.

4. The relationship between the intended use of the diagnostic test and the drug.

The utility of a diagnostic test relies on whether its ability to differentiate the clinical outcomes, either efficacy or safety, is better in the tested population than in the untested one. Therefore, another design that may be useful to test the overall benefit/risk of the drug-diagnostic test is first to randomly divide the patients into two groups: the tested group and the untested group. The patients in the untested group will not be given the diagnostic test and will be randomized to the drug or the concurrent control. Design B is then used for the tested group in which patients are stratified according to their results of the test for the molecular targets. This design allows us to investigate the difference in magnitude of the treatment effect between the tested positive group, tested negative group, and the untested group and hence to provide information about the utility of the diagnostic device.

5.3.3   Statistical Analyses

The U.S. FDA co-development concept paper (2005) pointed out that every effort should be made to verify the clinical hypothesis being claimed within a study that is independent from the analytical and clinical studies on which the diagnostic test was initially developed. In other words, the analytical performance of the diagnostic device should be based on the data that is independent and prior to the prospective or retrospective samples on which it is to be clinically verified. On the other hand, post hoc characterization of a diagnostic device based on the clinical utility data may be quite misleading, because the positive response observed in a subgroup of the patients determined by the threshold based on the clinical validation sample may be actually due to chance alone. In addition, the chance association increases when the number of features (genes) included in the diagnostic device increases.

Another issue of statistical analysis is to incorporate the diagnostic inaccuracy into estimation of the treatment effect in the patient population actually with the molecular targets. As demonstrated earlier, the PPV for the metastatic disease at 10 years of MammaPrint is only 29%. In addition, the area under the ROC curve of the 70-gene signature for predicting the OS at 10 years is only 0.648. As a result, for a diagnostic device with a very low PPV, a nonsignificant finding of chemotherapy does not imply that the drug is not effective in the patients truly with the molecular targets. This is because metastasis will not occur in 71% of patients tested positive, in which chemotherapy is unlikely to be beneficial and is very likely to be toxic.

Following the observations by Liu and Chow (2008), consider that there is a validated diagnostic device for a particular molecular target, a randomized trial to compare the test drug (T) with a concurrent control (C), and the primary endpoint is continuous. Table 5.3 provides the population means by treatment and diagnosis of the molecular target. In Table 5.3, μ_{T+}, $\mu_{C+}(\mu_{T-}, \mu_{C-})$ are the means of test and control groups for the patients with (without) the molecular target. Let $\overline{Y}_{T+}$ and $\overline{Y}_{C+}$ be the sample means of the test and control treatments, respectively, for the patients with a positive diagnosis of the molecular target. Since no diagnostic test is perfect for the correct diagnosis of the molecular target without error, the patients with a positive diagnosis still may not have the molecular target. It follows

$$E(\overline{Y}_{T+} - \overline{Y}_{C+}) = \lambda(\mu_{T+} - \mu_{C+}) + (1 - \lambda)(\mu_{T-} - \mu_{C-})$$

where λ is the PPV of the diagnostic device for the target. Therefore, the expected value of the difference in the sample means consists of two components. The first component is the treatment effect of the test drug in the patients with a positive diagnosis truly having the molecular target, and the second component is the treatment effect of the patients with a positive diagnosis but in fact without the molecular

TABLE 5.3: Population means by treatment and diagnosis.

		Molecular Target		
Diagnosis	**True Status**	**Test**	**Control**	**Difference**
+(P$_+$)	+(PPV)	μ_{T+}	μ_{C+}	$\mu_{T+} - \mu_{C+}$
	$-$(FP)	μ_{T-}	μ_{C-}	$\mu_{T-} - \mu_{C-}$
$-$(P$_-$)	+(FN)	μ_{T+}	μ_{C+}	$\mu_{T+} - \mu_{C+}$
	$-$(NPV)	μ_{T-}	μ_{C-}	$\mu_{T-} - \mu_{C-}$

Note: P$_+$ (P$_-$) positive (negative) prevalence rate; PPV, positive predictive value; NPV, negative predictive value; FP, false positive rate; FN, false negative rate.

target. If the test treatment is ineffective in the patients without the molecular target, it follows that $|\mu_{T+} - \mu_{C+}| > |\mu_{T-} - \mu_{C-}|$, and the difference in the sample means observed from the patients with a positive result underestimates the treatment effects of the test drug in the patients with the molecular target. Similarly, the expected value of the difference in the sample means between the test drug and concurrent control from the patients tested negative for the molecular target, $\overline{Y}_{T-} - \overline{Y}_{C-}$ is given as

$$E(\overline{Y}_{T-} - \overline{Y}_{C-}) = \tau(\mu_{T-} - \mu_{C-}) + (1 - \tau)(\mu_{T+} - \mu_{C+})$$

where τ is the NPV of the diagnostic device for the target.

It abides by the fact that the observed treatment difference in the patients with a negative result overestimates the treatment effect in the patients truly without the molecular targets. In addition, if $\overline{Y}_{TU} - \overline{Y}_{CU}$ is the observed difference between the drug and control groups in the untested patients, then

$$E(\overline{Y}_{TU} - \overline{Y}_{CU}) = p[\lambda(\mu_{T+} - \mu_{C+}) + (1 - \lambda)(\mu_{T-} - \mu_{C-})]$$
$$+ (1 - p)[\tau(\mu_{T-} - \mu_{C-}) + (1 - \tau)(\mu_{T+} - \mu_{C+})]$$

where p is the prevalence rate of the untested patients truly with the molecular target. EM algorithm or Bayesian methods can be applied to obtain the treatment effects for the patients truly with and without the molecular target and treatment-by-device interaction. These results in comparison with the observed treatment differences of the patients tested positive and negative, and untested patients will provide important information regarding the true utility of the diagnostic device.

5.4 Discussion

As pointed by Doroshow (2005), although amplification of gene numbers and over-expression of EGFR are associated with the response of the treatment of erlotinib, objective responses were still observed in the patients without increasing the number of gene copies or over-expression of EGFR. This may imply that some other unknown signing pathway may affect the effect of erlotinib. Therefore, multiple pathological pathways and molecular targets are involved with the disease. As a result, treatments or drugs are being developed for multiple molecular targets. For example, sorefenib is a multikinase inhibitor, which inhibits Raf kinase, vascular endothelial growth factor receptors (VEGFR) 1, 2, and 3, RET receptor tyrosine kinase, c-kit protein, platelet-derived growth-factor receptor β (PDGFRβ), and FMS-like tyrosine kinase. However, the issues of the design and analysis for the drug-device co-development for the multiple targets can be quite complex and require further research.

Most of the diagnostic devices for detection of the molecular targets require the tissue samples. Therefore, the time of obtaining the tissue is also very important in the diagnosis for the molecular targets (Doroshow, 2005). For example, the tissue samples can be taken from the initial surgery, initial or subsequent biopsies, before the start of the treatment for the patients. To control the effect of tumor size and time from diagnosis to first therapy on the results of the diagnostic assay, a standardized approach for collection of tissue samples must be prospectively described in the protocol and uniformly performed for all the patients enrolled in the targeted clinical trials. This is just an example of the importance for ensuring the quality of the diagnostic assays. Another important issue, as mentioned earlier, is that the predictive molecular assays must be validated before the targeted clinical trials are initiated.

Although the design issues of targeted clinical trials have been discussed quite extensively, little attention has been paid to the issue of inaccuracy of molecular diagnostic devices in the inference of the treatment effects (Maitournam and Simon, 2005; Simon and Maitournam, 2005). In addition, the prevalence of the molecular targets also should be considered in the analysis of the data from the targeted clinical trials. However, the analyses of data from a targeted clinical trial should address its objectives. Therefore, whether the results of the molecular assays is a covariate or is a stratification factor depends on the goals of the trials. On the other hand, especially during the drug-device co-development, the drug-device interaction and comparison of treatment effects between the tested and untested patients for the utility of the device may also be very important. Therefore, a great challenge lies ahead for the inference of the targeted clinical trials.

References

The ALTTO trial. 2008a http://www.cancer.gov/, accessed on March 1, 2008.

The ALTTO trial. 2008b http://www.clinincaltrial.gov, accessed on March 1, 2008.

The ALTTO trial. 2008c http://www.breastinternaitonalgroup.org, accessed on March 1, 2008.

Bazell, R. *Her-2: The Making of Herceptin, A Revolutionary Treatment for Breast Cancer.* Random House, New York, 1998.

Buyse, M., Loi, S., van't Veer, L., et al. 2006. Validation and clinical utility of a 70-gene prognostic signature for women with node-negative breast caner. *Journal of the National Cancer Institute* 98, 1183–1192.

Casciano, D.A. and Woodcock, J. 2006. Empowering microarrays in the regulatory setting. *Nature Biotechnology* 24, 1103.

Chow, S.C. and Liu, J.P. *Design and Analysis of Clinical Trials.* Wiley, New York, 2004.

Dalton, W.S. and Friend, S.H. 2006. Cancer biomarkers—An invitation to the table. *Science* 312, 1165–1168.

Demetri, G.D., von Mehren, M., Blanke, C.D., et al. 2002. Efficacy and safety of imatinib mesylate in advanced gastrointestinal stromal tumors, *New England Journal of Medicine*, 347, 472–480.

Doroshow, J.H. 2005. Targeting EGFR in non-small-cell-lung cell. *New England Journal of Medicine* 353, 200–202.

Druker, B.J., Talpaz, M., Resta, D.J., et al. 2001. Efficacy and safety of a specific inhibitor of the BCR-ABL tyrosine kinase in chronic myeloid leukemia. *New England Journal of Medicine* 344, 1031–1037.

Evans, W.E. and McLeod, H.L. 2003. Pharmacogenomics—drug disposition, drug targets, and side effects. *New England Journal of Medicine* 348, 538–549.

FDA Decision Summary P980018, Rockville, Maryland, 1998.

FDA Decision Summary P980024/S001, Rockville, Maryland, 2001.

FDA Decision Summary P040030, Rockville, Maryland, 2004.

FDA Draft concept paper on *Drug-Diagnostic Co-Development*, Rockville, Maryland, 2005.

FDA Annotated Redlined Draft Package Insert for Herceptin, Rockville, Maryland, 2006.

FDA Decision Summary k062694, Rockville, Maryland, 2007.

Fukuoka, M., Yano, S., Giaccone, G., et al. 2003. Multi-institutional randomized phase II trial of gefinib for previously treated patients with advanced non-small-cell lung cell. *Journal of Clinical Oncology* 21, 2237–2246.

Herbst, R.S., Giaccone, G., Schiller, J.H., et al. 2004. Gefitinib in combination with paclitaxel and carboplatin in advanced non-small-cell lung cancer, a phase III trial – INTACT 2. *Journal of Clinical Oncology* 22, 785–794.

Hortobagyi, G.N. 1998. Treatment of breast cancer. *New England Journal of Medicine* 329, 974–984.

Kantarjian, H., Sawyers, C., Hochhaus, A., et al. 2002. The International STI571 CML Study Group. Hematologic and cytogenetic responses to imatinib mesylate in chronic myelogenous leukemia. *New England Journal of Medicine* 346, 645–652.

Kris, M.G., Natale, R.B. Herbst, R.S., et al. 2003. Efficacy of gefitinib, an inhibitor of the epidermal growth factor receptor tyrosine kinase, in symptomatic patients with non-small cell lung cancer. *Journal of the American Medical Association* 290, 2149–2158.

Liu, J.P. and Chow, S.C. 2008. Statistical issues on the diagnostic multivariate index assay and targeted clinical trials. *Journal of Biopharmaceutical Statistics* 18, 167–182.

Maitournam, A. and Simon, R. 2005. On the efficiency of targeted clinical trials. *Statistics in Medicine* 24, 329–339.

MINDACT Design and MINDACT trial overview. 2008. http://www.breast internationalgroup.org/transbig.html. Accessed on February 20, 2008.

O'Brien, S.J. and Dean, M. 1997. In search of AIDS-resistance genes. *Scientific American* 277, 44–51.

Paik, S., Shak, S., Tang, G., et al. 2004. A multigene assay to predict recurrence of tamoxifen-treated, node-negative breast cancer. *New England Journal of Medicine* 351, 2817–2826.

Paik, S., Tang, G., Shak, S., et al. 2006. Gene expression and benefit of chemotherapy in women with node-negative, estrogen receptor-positive breast cancer. *Journal of Clinical Oncology* 24, 1–12.

Ravdin, P.M. and Chamness, G.C. 1995. The c-erbB-2 proto-oncogene as a prognostic and predictive markers in breast cancer: A paradigm for the development of other macromolecular markers—a review. *Gene* 159, 19–27.

Rubin, B.P., Singer, S., Tsao, C., et al. 1996. KIT activation is a ubiquitous feature of gastrointestinal stromal tumors. *Cancer Research* 61, 8118–8121.

Romond, E.H., Perez, E.A., Bryant, J. et al. 2005. Trastuzumab plus chemotherapy for operable HER2-positive breast cancer. *New England Journal of Medicine* 353, 1673–1684.

Seshadri, R., Figaira, F.A., Horsfall, D.J., et al. 1993. Clinical significance of HER-2/neu oncogene amplification in primary cancer. *Journal of Clinical Oncology* 11, 1936–1942.

Shepherd, F.A., Pereira, J.R., Ciuleanu, T., et al. 2005. Erlotinib in previously treated non-small-cell lung cancer. *New England Journal of Medicine* 353, 123–132.

Simon, R. and Maitournam, A. 2004. Evaluating the efficiency of targeted designs for randomized clinical trials. *Clinical Cancer Research* 10, 6759–6763.

Slamon, D.J., Leyland-Jones, B., Shak, S., et al. 2001. Use of chemotherapy plus a monoclonal antibody against HER2 for metastatic breast cancer that overexpresses HER2. *New England Journal of Medicine* 344, 783–792.

Sprarano, J., Hayes, D., Dees, E. et al. 2006. Phase III randomized study of adjuvant combination chemotherapy and hormonal therapy versus adjuvant hormonal therapy alone in women with previously resected axillary node-negative breast cancer with various levels of risk for recurrence (TAILORx Trial). http://www.cancer.gov/clinicaltrials/ECOG- PACCT-1, accessed on February 26, 2008.

Tsao, M.S., Sakurada, A., Cutz, J.C., et al. 2005. Erlotinib in lung cancer—molecular and clinical predictors of outcome. *New England Journal of Medicine* 353, 133–144.

van't Veer, L.J., Dai, H., van de Vijver, M.J., et al. 2002. Gene expression profiling predicts clinical outcome of breast cancer. *Nature* 415, 530–536.

Van de Vijver, M.J., He, Y.D., van't Veer, L.J., et al. 2002. A gene-expression signature as a predictor of survival in breast cancer. *New England Journal of Medicine* 347, 1999–2009.

Varmus, H. 2006. The new era in cancer research. *Science* 312, 1162–1165.

Weinshilboum, R. 2003. Inheritance and drug response. *New England Journal of Medicine* 348, 529–537.

Winkler, C., Modi, W., Smith M.W., et al. 1998. Genetic restriction of AIDS pathogenesis by an SDF-1 chemokine gene variant. *Science* 278:389–393.

Chapter 6

Statistical Methods in Translational Medicine

Shein-Chung Chow, Siu-Keung Tse, and Dennis Cosmatos

Contents

6.1 Introduction

As pointed out in Chapter 1, the United States Food and Drug Administration (FDA) kicked off the Critical Path Initiative in early 2000 to assist the sponsors in identifying the possible causes of scientific challenges underlying the medical product pipeline problems. The Critical Path Opportunities List released by the FDA on March 16, 2006 identified (1) better evaluation tools and (2) streamlining clinical trials as the top two topic areas to bridge the gap between the quick pace of new biomedical discoveries and the slower pace at which those discoveries are currently developed into therapies. This has led to the consideration of the use of adaptive design methods in clinical development and the focus of translational science/research, which attempt not only to identify the best clinical benefit of a drug product under investigation, but also try to increase the probability of success. Statistical methods for the use of adaptive trial designs in the clinical development can be found in Chow and Chang (2006) and Chang (2007). In this chapter, we will focus on the statistical methods that are commonly employed in translational science/research.

Chow (2007) classified translational science/research into three areas, namely, translation in language, translation in information, and translation in (medical) technology. Translation in language is referred to the possible lost in translation of inform consent form or case report forms in multinational clinical trials. Lost in translation is commonly encountered because of not only difference in language, but also differences in perception, culture, medical practices, etc. A typical approach for assessment of the possible lost in translation is to first translate the inform consent form or the case report forms by an experienced expert and then translate back by a different experienced but independent expert. The back-translated version is then compared with the original version for consistency. If the back-translated version passes the test for consistency, then the back-translated version is validated through a small-scale pilot study before it is applied to the intended multinational clinical trial. Translation in information is referred to as bench-to-bedside in translational science/research, which is also known as translational medicine (TM). Translation in technology includes biomarker development and translation in diagnostic procedures between traditional Chinese medicine and Western medicine. In this chapter, we will focus on the statistical methods for translation in information and translation in technology. It must be noted that in practice, TM is often divided into two areas, discovery TM and clinical TM. Discovery TM includes biomarker development, bench-to-bedside, and animal model versus human model, while clinical TM includes translation among study endpoints, translation in technology, and the generalization from one target patient population to another.

In the next section, statistical method for optimal variable screening in microarray analysis is outlined, along with the cross-validation method for model selection and validation. Section 6.3 discusses the statistical methods for the assessment of one-way/two-way translation and lost in translation in bench-to-bedside translational process in pharmaceutical development. Whether or not an established animal model is predictive of a human model is examined in Section 6.4. In Section 6.5, the relationships between different study endpoints, which are derived from data collected from the same target patient population, are discussed. Issues that are commonly encountered in translation in technology are described in Section 6.6. The generalization of the results obtained from one target patient population to another similar but different target patient population is discussed in Section 6.7. Finally, some concluding remarks are provided in the last section of this chapter.

6.2 Biomarker Development

Biomarker is a characteristic that is objectively measured and evaluated as an indicator of the normal biological processes, pathogenic process, or pharmacologic responses to a therapeutic intervention. Biomarkers can be classified into classifier marker, prognostic marker, and predictive marker. A classifier marker usually does not change over the course of study and can be used to identify the patient population who would be benefited from the treatment from those who do not. A typical example is a DNA marker for a population selection in the enrichment process of clinical trials. A prognostic marker informs the clinical outcomes, which is independent of the treatment. A predictive marker informs the treatment effect on the clinical endpoint, which could be population-specific, i.e., a predictive marker could be predictive for population A but not population B. It should be noted that the correlation between biomarker and true endpoint makes a prognostic marker. However, correlation between biomarker and true endpoint does not make a predictive biomarker.

In clinical development, a biomarker could be used to select the right population, identify the nature course of the disease, early detection of the disease, and help to develop personalized medicine. The utilization of biomarker could lead to a better target population, detection of a large effect size with smaller sample size, and a timely decision making. As indicated in the FDA Critical Path Initiative Opportunity List, better evaluation tools call for biomarker qualification and standards. Statistical methods for early-stage biomarker qualification include, but are not limited to (1) distance-dependent K-nearest neighbors (DD-KNN), (2) K means clustering, (3) single/average/complete linkage clustering, and (4) distance-dependent Jarvis–Patrick clustering. More information with respect to these can be found at http://www.ncifcrf.gov/human_studies.shtml.

In what follows, we will review the statistical methods that are commonly used in the biomarker development for optimal variable screening. The selected variables will then be used to establish a predictive model through a model selection/validation process.

6.2.1 Optimal Variable Screening

DNA microarrays have been used extensively in medicine practice. Microarrays identify a set of candidate genes that are possibly related to a clinical outcome of a disease (in disease diagnoses) or a medical treatment. However, there are much more candidate genes than the number of available samples (the sample size) in almost all the studies, which leads to an irregular statistical problem in the disease diagnoses or treatment-outcome prediction. Some available statistical methods deal with a single gene at a time (e.g., Chen and Chen, 2003), which clearly do not provide the best solution for polygenic diseases. In practice, meta analysis and/or combining several similar studies is often considered to increase sample size. These approaches, however, may not be appropriate owing to the fact that (1) the combined data set may still be much too small, and (2) there may be heteroscedasticity among the data from different studies. Alternatively, Shao and Chow (2007) proposed an optimal variable screening approach for dealing with the situation where the number of variables (genes) is much larger than the sample size.

Let y be a clinical outcome of interest and x be a vector of p candidate genes that are possibly related to y. Shao and Chow (2007) simply considered the inference on the population of y conditional on x and noted that their proposed method can be applied to the unconditional analysis (i.e., both y and x are random). Consider the following model

$$y = \beta'x + \varepsilon, \tag{6.1}$$

where β is a p-dimensional vector and the distribution of ε is independent of x with $E(\varepsilon) = 0$ and $E(\varepsilon^2) = \sigma^2$. Under the model (Equation 6.1), assume that there is a positive integer p_0 (which does not depend on n), such that only p_0 components of β are nonzero. Furthermore, β is in the linear space generated by the rows of $X'X$ for sufficiently large n, where X is the $n \times p_n$ matrix, whose ith row is x_i'. In addition, assume that there is a sequence $\{\xi_n\}$ of positive numbers such that $\xi_n \to \infty$ and $\lambda_{in} = b_i\xi_n$, where λ_{in} is the ith nonzero eigenvalue of $X'X, i = 1,\ldots,n$ and $\{b_i\}$ is a sequence of bounded positive numbers. Note that in many problems, $\xi_n = n$. Furthermore, there exists a constant $c > 0$ such that $p_n/\xi_n^c \to 0$. For the estimation of β, Shao and Chow (2007) considered the following ridge regression estimator:

$$\hat{\beta} = (X'X + h_nI_{p_n})^{-1}X'Y, \tag{6.2}$$

where $Y = (y_1,\ldots,y_n)'$, I_{p_n} is the identity matrix of order p_n and $h_n > 0$ is the ridge parameter. The bias and variance of $\hat{\beta}$ are given by

$$\text{bias}(\hat{\beta}) = E(\hat{\beta}) - \beta = -(h_n^{-1}X'X + I_{p_n})^{-1}\beta$$

and

$$\text{var}(\hat{\beta}) = \sigma^2(X'X + h_nI_{p_n})^{-1}X'X(X'X + h_nI_{p_n})^{-1}.$$

Let β_i and $\hat{\beta}_i$ be the ith component of β and $\hat{\beta}$, respectively. Under the assumptions as described earlier, we have $E(\hat{\beta}_i - \beta_i)^2 \to 0$ (i.e., $\hat{\beta}_i$ is consistent for β_i in the mean squared error) if h_n is suitably chosen. Thus, we have

$$\text{var}(\hat{\beta}) = \frac{\sigma^2}{h_n}\left(\frac{X'X}{h_n} + I_{p_n}\right)^{-1}\frac{X'X}{h_n}\left(\frac{X'X}{h_n} + I_{p_n}\right)^{-1}. \tag{6.3}$$

Hence, $\text{var}(\hat{\beta}_i) \to 0$ for all i as long as $h_n \to \infty$. Note that the analysis of the bias of $\hat{\beta}_i$ is more complicated. Let Γ be an orthogonal matrix such that

$$\Gamma'X'X\Gamma = \begin{pmatrix} \Lambda_n & 0_{n\times(p_n-n)} \\ 0_{(n-p_n)\times n} & 0_{(p_n-n)\times(p_n-n)} \end{pmatrix},$$

where Λ_n is a diagonal matrix whose ith diagonal element is λ_{in} and $0_{l\times k}$ is the $l \times k$ matrix of 0s. Then, it follows that

$$\text{bias}(\hat{\beta}) = -\left[\Gamma\left(\frac{\Gamma'X'X\Gamma}{h_n} + I_{p_n}\right)\Gamma'\right]^{-1}\beta = -\Gamma A\Gamma'\beta, \tag{6.4}$$

where A is a $p_n \times p_n$ diagonal matrix whose first n diagonal elements are

$$\frac{h_n}{h_n + \lambda_{in}}, \quad i = 1, \ldots, n,$$

and all the last diagonal elements are equal to 1. Under the above-mentioned assumptions, combining the results for variance and bias of $\hat{\beta}_i$, i.e., Equations 6.3 and 6.4, it can be shown that for all i

$$E(\hat{\beta}_i - \beta_i)^2 = \text{var}(\hat{\beta}_i) + \left[\text{bias}(\hat{\beta}_i)\right]^2 \to 0$$

if h_n is chosen so that $h_n \to \infty$ is at a rate slower than ξ_n (e.g., $h_n = \xi_n^{2/3}$). Based on this result, Shao and Chow (2007) proposed the following optimal variable screening procedure:

Let $\{a_n\}$ be a sequence of positive numbers satisfying $a_n \to 0$. For each fixed n, we screen out the ith variable if and only if $|\hat{\beta}_i| \leq a_n$.

Note that, after screening, only variables associated with $|\hat{\beta}_i| > a_n$ are retained in the model as predictors. The idea behind this variable screening procedure is similar to that in the Lasso method (Tibshirani, 1996). Under certain conditions, Shao and Chow (2007) showed that their proposed optimal variable screen method is consistent in the sense that the probability that all variables (genes) unrelated to y will be screened out, and all variables (genes) related to y will be retained as 1, as n tends to be infinity.

6.2.2 Model Selection and Validation

Consider that n data points are available for selecting a model from a class of models. Several methods for model selection are available in the literature. These methods include, but are not limited to, Akaike information criterion (AIC) (Akaike, 1974; Shibata, 1981), the C_p (Mallows, 1973), the jackknife, and the bootstrap (Efron, 1983, 1986). These methods, however, are not asymptotically consistent in the sense that the probability of selecting the model with the best predictive ability does not converge to 1 as the total number of observations $n \to \infty$. Alternatively, Shao (1993) proposed a method for model selection and validation using the method of cross-validation. The idea of cross-validation is to split the data set into two parts. The first part contains n_c data points, which will be used for fitting a model (model construction), whereas the second part contains $n_v = n - n_c$ data points, which are reserved for assessing the predictive ability of the model (model validation). It should be noted that all of the $n = n_c + n_v$ data, not just n_v are used for model validation. Shao (1993) demonstrated that all the methods of AIC, C_p, Jackknife, and bootstrap are asymptotically equivalent to the cross-validation with $n_v = 1$, denoted by CV(1), although they share the same deficiency of inconsistency. Shao (1993) indicated that the inconsistency of the leave-one-out cross-validation can be rectified by using leave-n_v-out cross-validation with n_v satisfying $n_v/n \to 1$ as $n \to \infty$.

In addition to the cross-validation with $n_v = 1$, denoted by CV(1), Shao (1993) also considered the other two cross-validation methods, namely, a Monte Carlo cross-validation with n_v ($n_v \neq 1$), denoted by MCCV(n_v), and an analytic approximate CV(n_v), denoted by APCV(n_v). MCCV(n_v) is a simple and easy method, utilizing the method of Monte Carlo by randomly drawing (with or without replacement) a collection $\mathfrak{R}$ of b subsets of $\{1, \ldots, n\}$ that have size n_v, and selecting a model by minimizing

$$\hat{\Gamma}_{\alpha,n} = \frac{1}{n_v b} \sum_{s \in \mathfrak{R}} \|y_s - \hat{y}_{\alpha,s^c}\|^2 .$$

On the other hand, APCV(n_v) selects the optimal model based on the asymptotic leading term of balance incomplete CV(n_v), which treats each subset as a block and each i as a treatment. Shao (1993) compared these three cross-validation methods through a simulation study under the following model with five variables with $n = 40$:

$$y_i = \beta_1 x_{1i} + \beta_2 x_{2i} + \beta_3 x_{3i} + \beta_4 x_{4i} + \beta_5 x_{5i} + e_i,$$

where are i.i.d. from $N(0,1)$, x_{ki} is the ith value of the kth prediction variable x_k, $x_{1i} = 1$, and the values of $x_{ki}, k = 2, \ldots, 5, i = 1, \ldots, 40$, are taken from an example in the work by Gunst and Mason (1980). Note that there are 31 possible models, and each model is denoted by a subset of $\{1, \ldots, 5\}$ that contains the indices of the variable x_k in the model. Shao (1993) indicated that MCCV(n_v) has the best performance among the three methods under study, except for the case where the largest model is the optimal model. APCV(n_v) is observed to be slightly better than the CV(1) in all cases. CV(1) tends to select unnecessarily large models. The probability of selecting the optimal model by using the CV(1) could be very low (e.g., <0.5).

6.2.3   Remarks

In practice, it is suggested that the optimal variable screening method proposed by Shao and Chow (2007) be applied to select a few relevant variables, say 5–10 variables. Then, the cross-validation method can be applied to select the optimal model, based on linear (Shao, 1993) or nonlinear model selection (Li, Chow, and Smith, 2004). The selected model can then be validated based on the cross-validation methods as described in Section 6.2.2.

6.3   Bench-to-Bedside

Pizzo (2006) defined TM as "bench-to-bedside" research, wherein a basic laboratory discovery becomes applicable to the diagnosis, treatment, or prevention of a specific disease, brought forth either by a physician-scientist, who works at the interface between the research laboratory and patient care, or by a team of basic and clinical science investigators. Thus, TM is referred to the translation of basic research discoveries into clinical applications. More specifically, TM takes the discoveries from basic research to a patient and measures an endpoint in a patient. Most recently, scientists are increasingly becoming aware that this bench-to-bedside approach to translational research is a two-way street. Basic scientists provide clinicians with new tools for use in patients and for assessment of their impact, while clinical researchers make novel observations about the nature and progression of the disease that often stimulate basic investigations. As indicated by Pizzo (2006), TM can also have a much broader definition, referring to the development and application of new technologies, biomedical devices, and therapies in a patient-driven environment, such as clinical trials, where the emphasis is on early patient testing and evaluation. Thus, TM also includes epidemiological and health-outcome researches and behavioral studies that can be brought to the bedside or ambulatory setting.

Mankoff et al. (2004) pointed out that there are three major obstacles to effective TM in practice. The first is the challenge of translating basic science discoveries into clinical studies. The second hurdle is the translation of clinical studies into medical practice and healthcare policy. The third obstacle to effective TM is philosophical. It may be a mistake to think that basic science (without observations from the clinical study and without epidemiological findings of possible associations between different diseases) will efficiently produce the novel therapies for human testing. Pilot studies, such as nonhuman and nonclinical studies, are often used to transition therapies developed using animal models to a clinical setting. Statistical process plays an important role in TM. In this chapter, we define a statistical process of TM as a translational process for (1) determining the association between some independent parameters observed in basic research discoveries and a dependent variable observed from clinical application, (2) establishing a predictive model between the independent parameters and the dependent response variable, and (3) validating the established predictive model. For example, in animal studies, the independent variables may include *in vitro* assay results, pharmacological activities such as pharmacokinetics (PKs) and pharmacodynamics (PDs), and dose toxicities, and the dependent variable could be a clinical outcome (e.g., a safety parameter).

6.3.1 One-Way Translation

Let x and y be the observed values from basic research discoveries and clinical application, respectively. In practice, it is important to ensure that the translational process is accurate and reliable with some statistical assurance. One of the statistical criteria is to examine the closeness between the observed response y and the predicted response $\hat{y}$ via a translational process. To study this, we will first study the association between x and y and build up a model. Then, we must validate the model based on some criteria. For simplicity, we assume that x and y can be described by the following linear model:

$$y = \beta_0 + \beta_1 x + \varepsilon, \tag{6.5}$$

where ε follows a normal distribution with mean 0 and variance σ_e^2.

Consider that n pairs of observations $(x_1, y_1), \ldots, (x_n, y_n)$ are observed in a translation process. To define notation, let

$$X^T = \begin{pmatrix} 1 & 1 & \cdots & 1 \\ x_1 & x_2 & \cdots & x_n \end{pmatrix} \quad \text{and} \quad Y^T = \begin{pmatrix} y_1 & y_2 & \cdots & y_n \end{pmatrix}.$$

Then, with respect to Equation 6.5, the maximum likelihood estimates (MLEs) of the parameters β_0 and β_1 can be given as

$$\begin{pmatrix} \hat{\beta}_0 \\ \hat{\beta}_1 \end{pmatrix} = (X^T X)^{-1} X^T Y$$

with

$$\text{var} \begin{pmatrix} \hat{\beta}_0 \\ \hat{\beta}_1 \end{pmatrix} = (X^T X)^{-1} \sigma_e^2.$$

Thus, we have established the following relationship:

$$\hat{y} = \hat{\beta}_0 + \hat{\beta}_1 x. \tag{6.6}$$

For the given x_i, from Equation 6.6 the corresponding fitted value $\hat{y}_i$ is $\hat{y}_i = \hat{\beta}_0 + \hat{\beta}_1 x_i$. Furthermore, the corresponding MLE of σ_e^2 is $\hat{\sigma}_e^2 = \frac{1}{n} \sum_{i=1}^{n} (y_i - \hat{y}_i)^2 = \frac{n-2}{n} \text{MSE}$, where MSE is the mean squared errors of the fitted model.

For a given $x = x_0$, consider that the corresponding observed value is given by y; using Equation 6.6, the corresponding fitted value can be obtained as $\hat{y} = \hat{\beta}_0 + \hat{\beta}_1 x_0$. Note that $E(\hat{y}) = \beta_0 + \beta_1 x_0 = \mu_0$ and

$$\text{var}(\hat{y}) = \begin{pmatrix} 1 & x_0 \end{pmatrix} (X^T X)^{-1} \begin{pmatrix} 1 \\ x_0 \end{pmatrix} \sigma_e^2 = c\sigma_e^2,$$

where $c = \begin{pmatrix} 1 & x_0 \end{pmatrix} (X^T X)^{-1} \begin{pmatrix} 1 \\ x_0 \end{pmatrix}$. Furthermore, $\hat{y}$ is normally distributed with mean μ_0 and variance $c\sigma_e^2$, i.e., $\hat{y} \sim N(\mu_0, c\sigma_e^2)$.

We may validate the translation model by considering the closeness of an observed y and its predicted value $\hat{y}$, obtained based on the fitted regression model given by Equation 6.6. To assess the closeness, we propose the following two measures, which are based on either the absolute difference or the relative difference between y and $\hat{y}$:

Criterion I. $p_1 = P\{|y - \hat{y}| < \delta\}$,

Criterion II. $p_2 = P\left\{ \left| \dfrac{y - \hat{y}}{y} \right| < \delta \right\}$.

In other words, it is desirable to have a high probability that the difference or the relative difference between y and $\hat{y}$, given by p_1 and p_2, respectively, is lesser than a clinically or scientifically meaningful difference δ. Then, for either $i = 1$ or 2, it is of interest to test the following hypotheses:

$$H_0: p_i \leq p_0 \quad \text{versus} \quad H_a: p_i > p_0, \tag{6.7}$$

where p_0 is some prespecified constant. If the conclusion is to reject H_0 in favor of H_a, this would imply that the established model is considered as validated. The technical details of the test of hypothesis corresponding to the two criteria are outlined in the following sections.

6.3.1.1 Test of Hypothesis for the Measures of Closeness

1. Measure of closeness based on absolute difference

Note that y and $\hat{y}$ are independent, thus $(y - \hat{y}) \sim N\left(0, (1+c)\sigma_e^2\right)$. It is easy to show that $p_1 = \Phi\left(\frac{\delta}{\sqrt{(1+c)\sigma_e^2}}\right) - \Phi\left(\frac{-\delta}{\sqrt{(1+c)\sigma_e^2}}\right)$. Thus, the MLE of p_1 is given by

$$\hat{p}_1 = \Phi\left(\frac{\delta}{\sqrt{(1+c)\,\hat{\sigma}_e^2}}\right) - \Phi\left(\frac{-\delta}{\sqrt{(1+c)\,\hat{\sigma}_e^2}}\right).$$

Using delta rule, for sufficiently large sample size n,

$$\text{var}\,(\hat{p}_1) = \left(\phi\left(\frac{\delta}{\sqrt{(1+c)\,\sigma_e^2}}\right) + \phi\left(\frac{-\delta}{\sqrt{(1+c)\,\sigma_e^2}}\right)\right)^2 \frac{\delta^2}{2(1+c)\,n\sigma_e^2} + o\left(\frac{1}{n}\right),$$

where $\phi(z)$ is the probability density function of a standard normal distribution. Furthermore, $\text{var}(\hat{p}_1)$ can be estimated by V_1, where V_1 is given by

$$V_1 = \frac{2\delta^2}{(1+c)\,n\hat{\sigma}_e^2}\phi^2\left(\frac{\delta}{\sqrt{(1+c)\,\hat{\sigma}_e^2}}\right).$$

Using Sluksty theorem, $\frac{\hat{p}_1 - p_0}{\sqrt{V_1}}$ can be approximated by a standard normal distribution. For testing the hypotheses $H_0: p_1 \le p_0$ versus $H_a: p_1 > p_0$, H_0 is rejected if $\frac{\hat{p}_1 - p_0}{\sqrt{V_1}} > z_{1-\alpha}$, where $z_{1-\alpha}$ is the $100(1-\alpha)$th percentile of a standard normal distribution.

2. Measure of closeness based on the absolute relative difference

Note that $\frac{y^2}{\sigma_e^2}$ and $\frac{\hat{y}^2}{c\sigma_e^2}$ follow a noncentral χ_1^2 distribution with noncentrality parameter μ_0^2/σ_e^2 and $\mu_0^2/c\sigma_e^2$, respectively, where $\mu_0 = \beta_0 + \beta_1 x_0$. Hence, $\frac{\hat{y}^2}{cy^2}$ is doubly noncentral F-distributed with $v_1 = 1$ and $v_2 = 1$ degrees of freedom and noncentrality parameters $\lambda_1 = \mu_0^2/c\sigma_e^2$ and $\lambda_2 = \mu_0^2/\sigma_e^2$. From the findings of Johnson and Kotz (1970), a noncentral F-distribution with v_1 and v_2 degrees of freedom can be approximated by $\frac{1+\lambda_1 v_1^{-1}}{1+\lambda_2 v_2^{-1}}F_{v,v'}$ where $F_{v,v'}$ is a central F-distribution with degrees of freedom $v = \frac{(v_1+\lambda_1)^2}{v_1+2\lambda_1} = \frac{(1+\mu_0^2/c\sigma_e^2)^2}{1+2\mu_0^2/c\sigma_e^2}$ and $v' = \frac{(v_2+\lambda_2)^2}{v_2+2\lambda_2} = \frac{(1+\mu_0^2/\sigma_e^2)^2}{1+2\mu_0^2/\sigma_e^2}$. Thus,

$$p_2 = P\left\{\left|\frac{y-\hat{y}}{y}\right| < \delta\right\}$$

$$= P\left\{\frac{(1-\delta)^2}{c} < \frac{\hat{y}^2}{cy^2} < \frac{(1+\delta)^2}{c}\right\}$$

$$\simeq P\left\{\frac{(1-\delta)^2}{c} < \frac{1+\lambda_1}{1+\lambda_2}F_{v,v'} < \frac{(1+\delta)^2}{c}\right\}$$

$$= P\left\{\frac{(1-\delta)^2}{c}\frac{1+\lambda_2}{1+\lambda_1} < F_{v,v'} < \frac{1+\lambda_2}{1+\lambda_1}\frac{(1+\delta)^2}{c}\right\}$$

Accordingly, p_2 can be estimated by

$$\hat{p}_2 = P\left\{\frac{(1-\delta)^2}{c}\frac{1+\hat{\lambda}_2}{1+\hat{\lambda}_1} < F_{\hat{v},\hat{v}'} < \frac{1+\hat{\lambda}_2}{1+\hat{\lambda}_1}\frac{(1+\delta)^2}{c}\right\} = P\left\{u_1 < F_{\hat{v},\hat{v}'} < u_2\right\},$$

where $u_1 = \frac{(1+\hat{\lambda}_2)}{c(1+\hat{\lambda}_1)}(1-\delta)^2$, $u_2 = \frac{(1+\hat{\lambda}_2)}{c(1+\hat{\lambda}_1)}(1+\delta)^2$, and $\left(\hat{\lambda}_1,\hat{\lambda}_2,\hat{v},\hat{v}'\right)$ are the corresponding MLE of $(\lambda_1,\lambda_2,v,v')$.

For a sufficiently large sample size, using Sluksty theorem, $\hat{p}_2$ can be approximated by a normal distribution with mean p_2 and variance V_2, where

$$V_2 = \left(\frac{\partial\hat{p}_2}{\partial\hat{\beta}_0},\frac{\partial\hat{p}_2}{\partial\hat{\beta}_1},\frac{\partial\hat{p}_2}{\partial\hat{\sigma}_e^2}\right)\begin{pmatrix} (X^TX)^{-1}\hat{\sigma}_e^2 & 0 \\ 0' & \frac{2\hat{\sigma}_e^4}{n-2} \end{pmatrix}\begin{pmatrix} \frac{\partial\hat{p}_2}{\partial\hat{\beta}_0} \\ \frac{\partial\hat{p}_2}{\partial\hat{\beta}_1} \\ \frac{\partial\hat{p}_2}{\partial\hat{\sigma}_e^2} \end{pmatrix};$$

with

$$\frac{\partial\hat{p}_2}{\partial\hat{\beta}_0} = \frac{2(c-1)\hat{\mu}_0}{c^2\hat{\sigma}_e^2(1+\hat{\lambda}_1)^2}\left[(1+\delta)^2 f_{\hat{v},\hat{v}'}(u_2) - (1-\delta)^2 f_{\hat{v},\hat{v}'}(u_1)\right]$$

$$+ \frac{4\hat{\lambda}_1^2(1+\hat{\lambda}_1)}{\hat{\mu}_0(1+2\hat{\lambda}_1)^2}\int_{u_1}^{u_2}\frac{\partial f_{\hat{v},\hat{v}'}(x)}{\partial\hat{v}}dx + \frac{4\hat{\lambda}_2^2(1+\hat{\lambda}_2)}{\hat{\mu}_0(1+2\hat{\lambda}_2)^2}\int_{u_1}^{u_2}\frac{\partial f_{\hat{v},\hat{v}'}(x)}{\partial\hat{v}'}dx;$$

$$\frac{\partial\hat{p}_2}{\partial\hat{\beta}_1} = x_0\frac{\partial\hat{p}_2}{\partial\hat{\beta}_0};$$

$$\frac{\partial\hat{p}_2}{\partial\hat{\sigma}_e^2} = \frac{\hat{\lambda}_1 - \hat{\lambda}_2}{c\hat{\sigma}_e^2(1+\hat{\lambda}_1)^2}\left[(1+\delta)^2 f_{\hat{v},\hat{v}'}(u_2) - (1-\delta)^2 f_{\hat{v},\hat{v}'}(u_1)\right]$$

$$- \frac{2\hat{\lambda}_1^2(1+\hat{\lambda}_1)}{\hat{\sigma}_e^2(1+2\hat{\lambda}_1)^2}\int_{u_1}^{u_2}\frac{\partial f_{\hat{v},\hat{v}'}(x)}{\partial\hat{v}}dx - \frac{2\hat{\lambda}_2^2(1+\hat{\lambda}_2)}{\hat{\sigma}_e^2(1+2\hat{\lambda}_2)^2}\int_{u_1}^{u_2}\frac{\partial f_{\hat{v},\hat{v}'}(x)}{\partial\hat{v}'}dx;$$

where $\frac{\partial f_{\hat{v},\hat{v}'}(x)}{\partial \hat{v}} = \frac{1}{2}f_{\hat{v},\hat{v}'}(x)\left[(\log\Gamma(\hat{v}+\hat{v}'))^{(1)} - (\log\Gamma(\hat{v}))^{(1)} + \log\left(\frac{\hat{v}x}{\hat{v}x+\hat{v}'}\right) + \frac{\hat{v}'(1-x)}{\hat{v}x+\hat{v}'}\right]$, $\frac{\partial f_{\hat{v},\hat{v}'}(x)}{\partial \hat{v}'} = \frac{1}{2}f_{\hat{v},\hat{v}'}(x)\left[(\log\Gamma(\hat{v}+\hat{v}'))^{(1)} - (\log\Gamma(\hat{v}'))^{(1)} + \log\left(\frac{\hat{v}'}{\hat{v}x+\hat{v}'}\right) - \frac{\hat{v}(1-x)}{\hat{v}x+\hat{v}'}\right]$ and $(\log\Gamma(s))^{(1)}$ is the first-order derivative of the natural logarithm of the gamma function with respect to s.

Thus, the hypotheses given in Equation 6.7 for one-way translation based on the probability of relative difference can be tested. In particular, H_0 is rejected if

$$Z = \frac{\hat{p}_2 - p_0}{\sqrt{V_2}} > z_{1-\alpha},$$

where $z_{1-\alpha}$ is the $100(1-\alpha)$th percentile of a standard normal distribution. Note that V_2 is an estimate of $\text{var}(\hat{p}_2)$, which is obtained by simply replacing the parameters with their corresponding estimates of the parameters.

6.3.1.2   Example 1

For the two measures proposed in Section 6.1, p_1 is based on the absolute difference between y and $\hat{y}$. For the given α, p_0, and the selected observation (x_0,y_0), the hypothesis $H_0: p_1 \leq p_0$ is rejected in favor of $H_a: p_1 > p_0$ when $Z = \frac{\hat{p}_1 - p_0}{\sqrt{V_1}} > z_{1-\alpha}$. Equivalently, H_0 is rejected if $(\hat{p}_1 - p_0 - z_{1-\alpha}\sqrt{V_1}) > 0$. Note that the value of $\hat{p}_1$ depends on the value of δ and it can be shown that $(\hat{p}_1 - p_0 - z_{1-\alpha}\sqrt{V_1})$ is an increasing function of δ over $(0, \infty)$. Thus, $(\hat{p}_1 - p_0 - z_{1-\alpha}\sqrt{V_1}) > 0$ only if $\delta > \delta_0$. Thus, the hypothesis H_0 can be rejected based on δ_0 instead of $\hat{p}_1$ as long as we can find the value of δ_0 for the given x_0. On the other hand, from a practical point of view, p_2 is more intuitive to understand, because it is based on the relative difference, which is equivalent to measure the percentage difference relative to the observed y, and δ can be viewed as the upper bound of the percentage error.

For illustration purpose, consider that the following data are observed in a translational study, where x is a given dose level and y is the associated toxicity measure:

x	0.9	1.1	1.3	1.5	2.2	2.0	3.1	4.0	4.9	5.6
y	0.9	0.8	1.9	2.1	2.3	4.1	5.6	6.5	8.8	9.2

When this set of data is fitted to Equation 6.5, the estimates of the equation parameters are given by $\hat{\beta}_0 = -0.704, \hat{\beta}_1 = 1.851, \hat{\sigma}^2 = 0.431$. Thus, based on the fitted results, given $x = x_0$, the proposed translation model is given by $\hat{y} = -0.704 + 1.851x_0$.

In this study, $\alpha = 0.05$ and $p_0 = 0.8$ were chosen. In particular, two dose levels $x_0 = 1.0$ and 5.2 were considered. Based on the study, the corresponding toxicity measures y_0 are 1.2 and 9.0, respectively. However, based on the translation model, the predicted toxicity measures are 1.147 and 8.921, respectively. In the following, the validity of the translation model is assessed by the two proposed closeness measures p_1 and p_2, respectively. Without loss of generality, $\alpha = 0.05$ and $p_0 = 0.8$ were chosen.

Case 1:   Testing of H_0: $p_1 \leq p_0$ versus H_a: $p_1 > p_0$

Using the above results, for $x_0 = 1.0$, δ is 1.112, since $|y_0 - \hat{y}| = |1.2 - 1.147| = 0.053$, which is less than $\delta = 1.112$, H_0 is rejected. Similarly, for $x_0 = 5.2$, the corresponding δ is 1.178, hence, $|y_0 - \hat{y}| = |9.0 - 8.921| = 0.079$, which is again smaller than $\delta = 1.178$, and thus H_0 is rejected.

Case 2:   Testing of H_0: $p_2 \leq p_0$ versus H_a: $p_2 > p_0$

Consider that $\delta = 1$ for the given two values of x, the estimates of p_2 and the corresponding values of the test statistic Z are given in the following table:

x_0	y_0	$\hat{y}$	$\hat{p}_2$	Z	Conclusion
1.0	1.2	1.147	0.870	1.183	Do not reject H_0
5.2	9.0	8.921	0.809	1.164	Do not reject H_0

6.3.2   Two-Way Translation

6.3.2.1   Validation of a Two-Way Translation Process

The above translational process is usually referred to as a "one-way translation" in TM, i.e., the information observed at basic research discoveries is translated to the clinical study. As indicated by Pizzo (2006), the translational process should be a *two-way translation*. In other words, we can exchange x and y of Equation 6.5

$$x = \gamma_0 + \gamma_1 y + \varepsilon$$

and come up with another predictive model $\hat{x} = \hat{\gamma}_0 + \hat{\gamma}_1 y$.

Following similar ideas, using either one of the measures p_i, the validation of a two-way translational process can be summarized by the following steps:

Step 1: For a given set of data (x, y), establish a predictive model, say, $y = f(x)$.

Step 2: Select the bound δ_{yi} for the difference between y and $\hat{y}$ Evaluate $\hat{p}_{yi} = P\{|y - \hat{y}| < \delta_{yi}\}$. Assess the one-way closeness between y and $\hat{y}$ by testing the hypotheses Equation 6.7. Proceed to the next step if the one-way translation process is validated.

Step 3: Consider x as the dependent variable and y as the independent variable. Set up the regression model. Predict x at the selected observation y_0, denoted by $\hat{x}$, based on the established model between x and y (i.e., $x = g(y)$), i.e., $\hat{x} = g(y) = \hat{\gamma}_0 + \hat{\gamma}_1 y$.

Step 4: Select the bound δ_{xi} for the difference between x and $\hat{x}$. Evaluate the closeness between x and $\hat{x}$ based on a test for the following hypotheses:

$$H_0: p_i \leq p_0 \quad \text{versus} \quad H_1: p_i > p_0$$

where $p_i = P\left\{\left|\frac{y-\hat{y}}{y}\right| < \delta_{yi} \text{ and } \left|\frac{x-\hat{x}}{x}\right| < \delta_{xi}\right\}$.

The above test can be referred to as a test for two-way translation. If, in Step 4, H_0 is rejected in favor of H_1, this would imply that there is a two-way translation between x and y (i.e., the established predictive model is validated). However, the evaluation of p involves the joint distribution of $\frac{x-\hat{x}}{x}$ and $\frac{y-\hat{y}}{y}$, and an exact expression is not readily available. Thus, an alternative approach is to modify Step 4 of the above-mentioned procedure and proceed with a conditional approach instead. In particular,

Step 4 (modified): Select the bound δ_{xi} for the difference between x and $\hat{x}$. Evaluate the closeness between x and $\hat{x}$ based on a test for the following hypotheses:

$$H_0: p_{xi} \le p_0 \quad \text{versus} \quad H_a: p_{xi} > p_0 \tag{6.8}$$

where $p_{xi} = P\{|x - \hat{x}| < \delta_{xi}\}$.

Note that the evaluation of p_{xi} is much easier and can be computed in a similar way by interchanging the role of x and y for the results given in Section 6.3.1.1.

6.3.2.2 Example 2

Using the data set given in Section 6.3.1.2, we set up the regression model $x = \gamma_0 + \gamma_1 y + \varepsilon$ with y as the independent variable and x as the dependent variable. The estimates of the model parameters are $\hat{\gamma}_0 = 0.468, \hat{\gamma}_1 = 0.519$, and $\hat{\sigma}^2 = 0.121$. Based on this model, for the same α and p_0, for the given $(x_0, y_0) = (1.0, 1.2)$ and $(5.2, 9.0)$, the fitted values are given by $\hat{x} = 0.468 + 0.519 y_0$.

Case 1: Testing of $H_0: p_{x1} \le p_0$ versus $H_a: p_{x1} > p_0$

Using the above results, for $y_0 = 1.2$, δ is 0.587, since $|x_0 - \hat{x}| = |1.0 - 1.09| = 0.09$, which is less than $\delta_x = 0.587$, H_0 is rejected. Similarly, for $y_0 = 9.0$, the corresponding δ is 0.624, then $|x_0 - \hat{x}| = |5.2 - 5.139| = 0.061$, which is again smaller than $\delta = 0.624$, and thus H_0 is rejected.

Case 2: Testing of $H_0: p_{x2} \le p_0$ versus $H_a: p_{x2} > p_0$

Suppose that $\delta = 1$, for the given two values of y, estimates of p_{x2} and the corresponding values of the test statistic Z are given in the following table:

x_0	y_0	$\hat{x}_0$	$\hat{p}_{x2}$	Z	Conclusion
1.0	1.2	1.090	0.809	1.300	Do not reject H_0
5.2	9.0	5.139	0.845	16.53	Do not reject H_0

6.3.3 Lost in Translation

It can be noted that δ_y and δ_x can be viewed as the maximum bias (or possible lost in translation) from the one-way translation (e.g., from basic research discovery to clinic) and from the other way of translation (e.g., from clinic to basic research discovery), respectively. If δ_y and δ_x given in Steps 2 and 4 of Section 6.3.2 are close to 0 with a relatively high probability, then we can conclude that the information from the basic research discoveries (clinic) is fully translated to clinic (basic research discoveries). Thus, one may consider the following parameter to measure the degree of lost in translation

$$\zeta = 1 - p_{xy}p_{yx},$$

where p_{xy} is the measure of closeness from x to y and p_{yx} is the measure of closeness from y to x. When $\zeta \approx 0$, we consider that there is no lost in translation. Overall lost in translation could be significant, even if the lost in translation from the one-way translation is negligible. For illustration purpose, if there is a 10% lost in translation in one-way translation and 20% lost in translation in the other way, there would be an up to 28% lost in translation. In practice, an estimate of ζ can be obtained for a given set of data (x,y). In particular, $\hat{\zeta} = 1 - \hat{p}_{xy}\hat{p}_{yx}$.

As an illustration, consider the example discussed in Section 6.3.1.2. Suppose that the measure of closeness based on relative difference is used, given $(x_0,y_0) = (1.0,1.2)$ and $(5.2, 9.0)$, the corresponding lost in translation for the two-way translation with $\delta = 1$ is tabulated in the following table:

x_0	y_0	$\hat{y}$	$\hat{p}_{xy}$	$\hat{x}$	$\hat{p}_{yx}$	$\hat{\zeta}$
1.0	1.2	1.147	0.870	1.090	0.809	0.296
5.2	9.0	8.921	0.809	5.139	0.845	0.316

6.4   Animal Model versus Human Model

In TM, a common question is whether an animal model is predictive of a human model. To address this question, we may assess the similarity between an animal model (population) and a human model (population). For this purpose, we first establish an animal model to bridge the basic research discovery (x) and clinic (y). For illustration purpose, consider one-way translation. Let $\hat{y} = \hat{\beta}_0 + \hat{\beta}_1 x$ be the predictive model obtained from the one-way translation based on data from an animal population. Thus, for a given x_0, $\hat{y}_0 = \hat{\beta}_0 + \hat{\beta}_1 x_0$, a distribution with mean μ_y and σ_y^2 is followed. Under the predictive model $\hat{y} = \hat{\beta}_0 + \hat{\beta}_1 x$, the target population is denoted by (μ_y,σ_y). Assume that the predictive model works for the target population. Thus, for an animal population, $\mu_y = \mu_{animal}$ and $\sigma_y = \sigma_{animal}$, while for a human population, $\mu_y = \mu_{human}$ and $\sigma_y = \sigma_{human}$. By assuming that the linear predictive model can be applied to both the animal and the human population, we can link the animal and human model by the following expressions:

$$\mu_{human} = \mu_{animal} + \varepsilon,$$

and

$$\mu_{human} = C\mu_{animal}.$$

In other words, we expect differences in population mean and standard deviation under the predictive model owing to possible difference in response between the animal and the human subjects. As a result, the effect size adjusted for standard deviation under the human population can be obtained as follows:

$$\left| \frac{\mu_{\text{human}}}{\sigma_{\text{human}}} \right| = \left| \frac{\mu_{\text{animal}} + \varepsilon}{C\sigma_{\text{animal}}} \right| = |\Delta| \left| \frac{\mu_{\text{animal}}}{\sigma_{\text{animal}}} \right|$$

where $\Delta = (1 + \varepsilon/\mu_{\text{animal}})/C$. Chow et al. (2002) referred to Δ as a sensitivity index when changing from one target population to another. As it can be observed, the effect size under the human population is inflated (or reduced) by the factor of Δ. If $\varepsilon = 0$ and $C = 1$, we then claim that there is no difference between the animal population and the human population. Thus, the animal model is predictive of the human model. Note that the shift and scale parameters (i.e., ε and C) can be estimated by

$$\hat{\varepsilon} = \hat{\mu}_{\text{human}} - \hat{\mu}_{\text{animal}}$$

and

$$\hat{C} = \frac{\hat{\sigma}_{\text{human}}}{\hat{\sigma}_{\text{animal}}},$$

respectively, in which $(\hat{\mu}_{\text{animal}}, \hat{\sigma}_{\text{animal}})$ and $(\hat{\mu}_{\text{human}}, \hat{\sigma}_{\text{human}})$ are estimates of $(\mu_{\text{animal}}, \sigma_{\text{animal}})$ and $(\mu_{\text{human}}, \sigma_{\text{human}})$, respectively. Thus, the sensitivity index can be assessed as follows:

$$\hat{\Delta} = (1 + \hat{\varepsilon}/\hat{\mu}_{\text{animal}})/\hat{C}.$$

In practice, there may be a shift in population mean (i.e., ε) or in population standard deviation (i.e., C). Chow et al. (2005) indicated that shifts in population mean and standard deviation can be classified into the following four cases: (1) both ε and C are fixed, (2) ε is random and C is fixed, (3) ε is fixed and C is random, and (4) both ε and C are random. For the case where both ε and C are fixed, $\hat{\Delta}$ can be used for estimation of Δ. Chow et al. (2005) derived statistical inference of Δ for the case where ε is random and C is fixed by assuming that y conditional on μ follows a normal distribution $N(\mu, \sigma^2)$. In other words,

$$y|_{\mu = \mu_{\text{human}}} \sim N(\mu, \sigma^2),$$

where μ is distributed as $N(\mu_\mu, \sigma_\mu^2)$ and σ, μ_μ, and σ_μ are some unknown constants. It can be verified whether y follows a mixed normal distribution with mean μ_μ and variance $\sigma^2 + \sigma_\mu^2$. That is, $y \sim N(\mu_\mu, \sigma^2 + \sigma_\mu^2)$. As a result, the sensitivity index can be assessed based on data collected from both animal and human population under the predictive model.

Note that for other cases where C is random, the above method can be derived similarly. The assessment of sensitivity index can be used to adjust the treatment effect to be detected under a human model when applying an animal model to a human model, especially when there is a significant or major shift between the animal and the human population. In practice, it is of interest to assess the impact of the sensitivity index on both lost in translation and the probability of success. This, however, requires further research.

6.5   Translation in Study Endpoints

In clinical trials, it is common that a study is powered based on expected absolute change from baseline of a primary study endpoint, but the collected data are analyzed based on relative change from baseline (e.g., percent change from baseline) of the primary study endpoint. In many cases, the collected data are analyzed based on the percentage of patients who show some improvement (i.e., responder analysis). The definition of a responder could be based on either absolute change from baseline or relative change from baseline of the primary study endpoint. It is very controversial in terms of the interpretation of the analysis results, especially when a significant result is observed based on a particular study endpoint (e.g., absolute change from baseline, relative change from baseline, or the responder analysis), but not on the other study endpoint. In practice, it is then of interest to explore how an observed significant difference of a study endpoint can be translated to that of the other study endpoint.

6.5.1   Power Analysis and Sample Size Calculation

An immediate impact on the assessment of treatment effect based on different study endpoints is the power analysis for sample size calculation. For example, sample size required to achieve the desired power, based on the absolute change could be very different from that obtained based on the percent change, or the percentage of patients who show an improvement based on the absolute change or relative change at α level of significance. Denote the measurements of the ith subject before and after the treatment by w_{1i} and w_{2i}, respectively. For illustration purpose, assume that w_{1i} are log-normal distributed, i.e., $\log w_{1i} \sim N(\mu_1, \sigma^2)$. Let $w_{2i} \equiv w_{1i}(\tilde{w}_{1i} + 1)$, where $\log \tilde{w}_{1i} \sim N(\mu_2, \sigma^2)$ and $w_{1i}, \tilde{w}_{1j}$ are independent for $1 \leq i$, $j \leq n$. It follows easily that $\log(w_{2i} - w_{1i}) \sim N(\mu_1 + \mu_2, 2\sigma^2)$ and $\log\left(\frac{w_{2i} - w_{1i}}{w_{1i}}\right) \sim N(\mu_2, \sigma^2)$. Define X_i and Y_i as $X_i = \log(w_{2i} - w_{1i})$, $Y_i = \log\left(\frac{w_{2i} - w_{1i}}{w_{1i}}\right)$. Thus, X_i and Y_i represent the logarithm of the absolute change and relative change of the measurements before and after the treatment. It can be shown that both X_i and Y_i are normally distributed. More details on the derivation of these results can be found in the Appendix.

Let μ_{AC} and μ_{RC} be the population means of the logarithm of the absolute change and relative change of a primary study endpoint of a given clinical trial, respectively. Thus, the hypotheses of interest based on the absolute change are given by

$$H_{01}: \mu_{AC} \leq \delta_0 \quad \text{versus} \quad H_{a1}: \mu_{AC} > \delta_0,$$

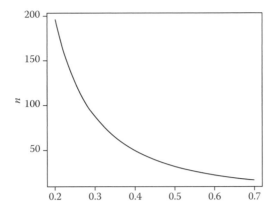

FIGURE 6.1: Plot of $(\delta - \delta_0)$ versus n.

where δ_0 is the difference of clinical importance. For the relative change, the hypotheses of interest are given by

$$H_{02}: \mu_{RC} \leq \Delta_0 \quad \text{versus} \quad H_{a2}: \mu_{RC} > \Delta_0,$$

where Δ_0 is the difference of clinical importance. In practice, a specific value of δ, for $\delta > \delta_0$, would be equivalent to that value of Δ with $\Delta > \Delta_0$ clinically. Figures 6.1 and 6.2 illustrate the plot of $(\delta - \delta_0)$ versus n (sample size) for a fixed desired power level 0.8, and plot of $(\Delta - \Delta_0)$ versus n (sample size) for a fixed desired power level 0.8, respectively, to provide a better understanding of their effects on the required sample size to achieve a targeted power level in testing the hypotheses H_{01} and H_{02}.

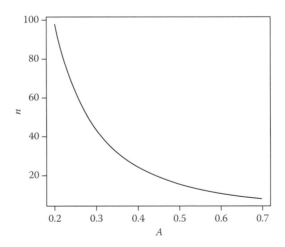

FIGURE 6.2: Plot of $(\Delta - \Delta_0)$ versus n.

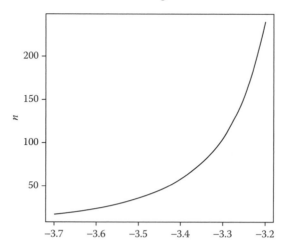

FIGURE 6.3:   Plot of ln δ versus n.

In addition, if we consider a patient as a responder if the logarithm of his/her absolute change of the primary study endpoint is $> \delta$, then, it is of interest to test the following hypotheses:

$$H_{03}: P_{AC} = \eta \quad \text{versus} \quad H_{a3}: P_{AC} > \eta,$$

where P_{AC} is the proportion of patients whose logarithm of the absolute change of the primary study endpoint is $> \delta$. In practice, we may claim superiority (clinically) of the test treatment if we reject the null hypothesis at $\eta = 50\%$ and favor the alternative hypothesis stating $P_{AC} > 50\%$. However, this lacks statistical justification. For a noninferiority (or superiority) trial, how the selection of a noninferiority margin of μ_{AC} can be translated to the noninferiority margin of P_{AC}? Similarly, for the relative change, the hypotheses of interest are given by

$$H_{04}: P_{RC} = \eta \quad \text{versus} \quad H_{a4}: P_{RC} > \eta,$$

where P_{RC} is the proportion of patients whose logarithm of the relative change of the primary study endpoint is $> \delta$. To provide a better understanding, Figures 6.3 and 6.4 provide the plots of δ versus n (sample size) for a fixed power level of 0.8 for the proportion, based on the absolute change and relative change, respectively. In particular, $\alpha = 0.05$ and $\eta = 0.5$.

Figures 6.3 and 6.4 show that the required sample size to achieve a desired power level can be very different depending on the type of endpoint adopted in the study.

6.5.2   Example 3

As an example, consider a clinical trial for the evaluation of possible weight reduction of a test treatment in female patients. Weight data from 10 subjects are given in Table 6.1. As it can be seen from Table 6.1, mean absolute change and mean percent

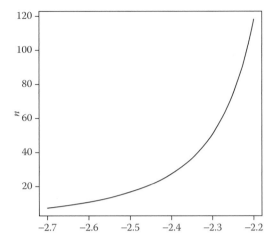

FIGURE 6.4: Plot of ln Δ versus *n*.

change from pretreatment are 5.3 lb and 4.8%, respectively. If a subject is considered a responder if there is weight reduction >5 lb (absolute change) or >5% (relative change), the response rates based on absolute change and relative change are given by 40% and 30%, respectively. For illustration purpose, Table 6.2 summarizes the sample sizes required for achieving a desired power for detecting a clinically meaningful difference, say, by an absolute change of 5.5 lb and a relative change of 5.5% for the two study endpoints, respectively.

As it can be seen from Table 6.2, a sample size of 190 are required for achieving an 80% power for detecting a difference of 5.5 lb (absolute change between posttreatment and pretreatment) at the 5% level of significance, while a much larger sample size of 95 is required to have an 80% power for detecting a difference of 5.5% (relative change between posttreatment and pretreatment) at the 5% level of significance. On the other hand, the results are different based on responder's

TABLE 6.1: Weight data from 10 female subjects.

Pretreatment	Posttreatment	Absolute Change	Relative Change (%)
110	106	4	3.6
90	80	10	11.1
105	100	5	4.8
95	93	2	2.1
170	163	7	4.1
90	84	6	6.7
150	145	5	3.3
135	131	4	3.0
160	159	1	0.6
100	91	9	9.0
Mean 120.5	115.2	5.3	4.8

TABLE 6.2:   Sample size calculation.

Study Endpoint	Clinical Meaningful Difference	Sample Size Required
Absolute change	5 lb	190
Relative change	5%	95
Responder 1[a]	50% improvement	54
Responder 2[b]	50% improvement	52

[a]   Responder is defined based on absolute change ≥ 5.5 lb.
[b]   Responder is defined based on relative change $\geq 5.5\%$.

analysis, where a total sample size of 54 subjects having ≥ 5.5 lb of weight reduction is needed for detecting a 50% improvement at the 5% level of significance. However, if we define a responder as a subject who has $\geq 5.5\%$ relative weight reduction, then a total sample size of 52 subjects is required for achieving a 50% improvement at the 5% level of significance.

6.5.3   Remarks

As discussed earlier, the sample sizes required for achieving a desired power for detecting a clinically meaningful difference at the 5% level of significance may be very different depending on (1) the choice of study endpoint and (2) the clinically meaningful difference. In practice, it will be more complicated if the intended trial is to establish noninferiority. In this case, sample size calculation will also depend on the selection of noninferiority margin. To ensure the success of the intended clinical trial, the sponsor will usually carefully evaluate several clinical strategies for selecting the type of study endpoint, clinically meaningful difference, and noninferiority margin during the stage of protocol development. The commonly considered study endpoints are

1. Measure based on absolute change

2. Measure based on relative change

3. Proportion of responders based on absolute change

4. Proportion of responders based on relative change

In some cases, some investigators may consider composite endpoint based on both absolute change and relative change. For example, in clinical trials for evaluation of the efficacy and safety of a compound for treating patients with active ulcerative colitis, a study endpoint utilizing the so-called Mayo score is often considered. The investigator may define a subject as a responder if he/she has a decrease of at least 3 points from the baseline in the total score and at least 30% with an accompanying decrease in the subscore of at least 1 point for rectal bleeding, or an absolute subscore of 0 or 1 for rectal bleeding on day 57. Note that Mayo scoring system for assessment of ulcerative colitis activity consists of three domains of (1) Mayo score, (2) partial Mayo score, and (3) mucosal healing (see, e.g., Rutgeerts et al., 2005).

In addition to the four types of study endpoints, which are derived from the clinical data collected from the sample patient population, clinically meaningful difference or noninferiority margin that we would like to detect or establish could be based on either absolute change or relative change. For example, based on the responder's analysis, we may want to detect a 30% difference or a 50% relative improvement in response rate. As a result, there are a total of eight clinical strategies for the assessment of the treatment effect. In practice, some strategies may lead to the success of the intended clinical trial (i.e., achieve the study objectives with the desired power), while some strategies may not. A common practice for the sponsor is to choose the strategy to their best interest. However, regulatory agencies may challenge the sponsor with respect to the inconsistent results. This has raised the following questions: (1) How to translate the clinical information among different study endpoints (since they are obtained based on the same data collected from certain patient population)? (2) Which study endpoint is accurate? However, till date, these questions still remain unanswered and further research is required to address these questions. Currently, the regulatory position is to necessitate the sponsor to prespecify the study endpoint that will be used for the assessment of the treatment effect in the study protocol, without any scientific justification.

6.6 Bridging Studies

In recent years, the influence of ethnic factors on clinical outcomes for evaluation of efficacy and safety of study medications under investigation has attracted much attention from regulatory authorities, especially when the sponsor is interested in bringing an approved drug product from the original region (e.g., the United States of America or European Union) to a new region (e.g., Asian Pacific Region). To determine if the clinical data generated from the original region are acceptable in the new region, the International Conference on Harmonization (ICH) issued a guideline on Ethnic Factors in the Acceptability of Foreign Clinical Data. The purpose of this guideline is not only to permit adequate evaluation of the influence of ethnic factors, but also to minimize duplication of clinical studies in the new region (ICH, 1998). This guideline is known as ICH E5 guideline.

As indicated in the ICH E5 guideline, a bridging study is defined as a study performed in the new region to provide PK, PD, or clinical data on the efficacy, safety, dosage, and dose regimen in the new region that will allow extrapolation of the foreign clinical data to the population in the new region. The ICH E5 guideline suggests the regulatory authority of the new region to assess the ability to extrapolate foreign data based on the bridging data package, which consists of (1) information including PK data and any preliminary PD, and dose-response data from the complete clinical data package (CCDP) that is relevant to the population of the new region, and (2) (if needed) bridging study to extrapolate the foreign efficacy data or safety data to the new region. The ICH E5 guideline indicates that bridging studies may not be necessary if the study medicines are insensitive to ethnic factors. For medicines characterized as insensitive to ethnic factors, the type of bridging studies (if needed) will depend on the experience with the drug class and the likelihood that extrinsic ethnic factors could affect the medicines' safety, efficacy, and dose-response. On the other hand, for medicines that are ethnically sensitive, bridging study is usually needed, since the populations in the two regions are different. In the ICH E5 guideline, however, no criteria for assessment of the sensitivity of the ethnic factors for determining whether a bridging study is needed are provided. Moreover, when a bridging study is conducted, the ICH guideline indicates that the study is readily interpreted as capable of bridging the foreign data, if it shows that dose-response, safety, and efficacy in the new region are similar to those in the original region. However, the ICH does not clearly define the similarity.

Shih (2001) interpreted it as the consistency among study centers by treating the new region as a new center of multicenter clinical trials. Under this definition, Shih (2001) proposed a method for assessment of consistency to determine whether the study is capable of bridging the foreign data to the new region. Alternatively, Shao and Chow (2002) proposed the concepts of reproducibility and generalizability probabilities for the assessment of bridging studies. If the influence of the ethnic factors is negligible, then we may consider the reproducibility probability to determine whether the clinical results observed in the original region are reproducible in the new region. If there is a notable ethnic difference, the generalizability probability can be assessed to determine whether the clinical results in the original region can be generalized in a similar but slightly different patient population, owing to the difference in the ethnic factors. In addition, Chow et al. (2002) assessed the bridging studies based on the concept of population (or individual) bioequivalence. Along this line, Hung (2003) and Hung et al. (2003) considered the assessment of similarity based on testing for noninferiority between a bridging study conducted in the new region and the previous study conducted in the original region. This leads to the argument regarding the selection of noninferiority margin (Chow and Shao, 2006). Note that other methods, such as the use of Bayesian approach, have also been proposed (see, e.g., Liu et al., 2002).

6.6.1 Test for Consistency

For assessment of similarity between a bridging study conducted in a new region and studies conducted in the original region, Shih (2001) considered all the studies conducted in the original region as a multicenter trial and proposed to test consistency among study centers by treating the new region as a new center of a multicenter trial.

Consider that there are K reference studies in the CCDP. Let T_i be the standardized treatment group difference, i.e.,

$$T_i = \frac{\bar{x}_{Ti} - \bar{x}_{Ci}}{s_i \sqrt{\frac{1}{m_{Ti}} + \frac{1}{m_{Ci}}}},$$

where $\bar{x}_{Ti}(\bar{x}_{Ci})$ is the sample mean of $m_{Ti}(m_{Ci})$ observations in the treatment (control) group, and s_i is the pooled sample standard deviation. Shih (2001) considered the following predictive probability for testing consistency:

$$p(T|T_i, i = 1,\ldots,K) = \left(\frac{2\pi(K+1)}{K}\right)^{-K/2} \exp\left[-K(T - \bar{T})^2/2(K+1)\right].$$

6.6.2 Test for Reproducibility and Generalizability

On the other hand, when the ethnic difference is negligible, Shao and Chow (2002) suggested assessing reproducibility probability for similarity between clinical results from a bridging study and studies conducted in the CCDP. Let x be a clinical response of interest in the original region. Let y be similar to x, but it is a response in a clinical bridging study conducted in the new region. Suppose the hypotheses of interest are

$$H_0: \mu_1 = \mu_0 \quad \text{versus} \quad H_a: \mu_1 \neq \mu_0.$$

We reject H_0 at the 5% level of significance only if $|T| > t_{n-2}$, where t_{n-2} is the $(1 - \alpha/2)$th percentile of the t distribution with $n - 2$ degrees of freedom, $n = n_1 + n_2$,

$$T = \frac{\bar{y} - \bar{x}}{\sqrt{\frac{(n_1-1)s_1^2+(n_0-1)s_0^2}{n-2}}\sqrt{\frac{1}{n_1} + \frac{1}{n_0}}},$$

and $\bar{x}, \bar{y}, s_0^2,$ and s_1^2 are sample means and variances for the original region and the new region, respectively. Thus, the power of T is given by

$$p(\theta) = P(|T| > t_{n-2}) = 1 - \Im_{n-2}(t_{n-2}|\theta) + \Im_{n-2}(-t_{n-2}|\theta),$$

where

$$\theta = \frac{\mu_1 - \mu_0}{\sigma\sqrt{\frac{1}{n_1} + \frac{1}{n_0}}},$$

and $\Im_{n-2}(\bullet|\theta)$ denotes the cumulative distribution function of the noncentral t-distribution with $n - 2$ degrees of freedom and the noncentrality parameter θ. Replacing θ in the power function with its estimate $T(x)$, the estimated power

$$\hat{p} = P(T(x)) = 1 - \Im_{n-2}(t_{n-2}|T(x)) + \Im_{n-2}(-t_{n-2}|T(x))$$

is defined as a reproducibility probability for a future clinical trial with the same patient population. Note that when the ethnic difference is notable, Shao and Chow (2002) recommended assessing the so-called generalizability probability for similarity between clinical results from a bridging study and studies conducted in the CCDP.

6.6.3   Test for Similarity

Using the criterion for assessment of population (individual) bioequivalence, Chow et al. (2002) proposed the following measure of similarity between x and y:

$$\theta = \frac{E(x-y)^2 - E(x-x')^2}{E(x-x')^2/2},$$

where x' is an independent replicate of x, and y, x, and x' are assumed to be independent. Since a small value of θ indicates that the difference between x and y is small (relative to the difference between x and x'), similarity between the new region and the original region can be claimed if and only if $\theta < \theta_U$, where θ_U is a similarity limit. Thus, the problem of assessing similarity becomes a problem of testing the following hypotheses:

$$H_0\colon \theta \geq \theta_U \quad \text{versus} \quad H_a\colon \theta < \theta_U.$$

Let $k = 0$ indicate the original region and $k = 1$ denote the new region. Consider that there are m_k study centers and n_k responses in each center for a given variable of interest. For simplicity, we only consider the balanced case where centers in a given region have the same number of observations. Let z_{ijk} be the ith observation from the jth center of region k, b_{jk} be the between-center random effect, and e_{ijk} be the within-center measurement error. Assume that

$$z_{ijk} = \mu_k + b_{jk} + e_{ijk}, \quad i = 1,\ldots,n_k, j = 1,\ldots,m_k, k = 0,1,$$

where μ_k is the population mean in region k, and $b_{jk} \sim N(0,\sigma_{Nk}^2), e_{ijk} \sim N(0,\sigma_{Wk}^2)$, and $\{b_{jk}\}$ and $\{e_{ijk}\}$ are independent. Under the above model, the criterion for similarity becomes

$$\theta = \frac{(\mu_0 - \mu_1)^2 + \sigma_{T1}^2 - \sigma_{T0}^2}{\sigma_{T0}^2},$$

where $\sigma_{Tk}^2 = \sigma_{Bk}^2 + \sigma_{Wk}^2$ is the total variance (between-center variance and within-center variance) in region k. The above hypotheses are equivalent to

$$H_0\colon \varsigma \geq 0 \quad \text{versus} \quad H_a\colon \varsigma < 0,$$

where $\varsigma = (\mu_0 - \mu_1)^2 + \sigma_{T1}^2 - (1 + \theta_U)\sigma_{T0}^2$.

6.7   Concluding Remarks

TM is a multidisciplinary entity that bridges the basic scientific research and clinical development. As the expense in developing therapeutic pharmaceutical compounds continues to increase and the success rates for getting such compounds approved for marketing and to the patients needing these treatments continues to decrease, a focused effort has emerged in improving the communication and planning between basic and clinical science. This will probably lead to more therapeutic insights being derived from the new scientific ideas, and more feedback being provided back to research so that their approaches are better targeted. TM spans all the disciplines and activities that lead to making key scientific decisions as a compound traverses across the difficult preclinical–clinical divide. Many argue that improvement in making correct decisions on what dose and regimen should be pursued in the clinic, the likely human safety risks of a compound, the likely drug interactions, and the pharmacologic behavior of the compound are probably the most important decisions made in the entire development process. Many of these decisions and the path for uncovering this information within later development are defined at this specific time within the drug development process. Improving these decisions will possibly lead to a substantial increase in the number of safe and effective compounds available to combat human diseases.

Appendix

Let w_{1i} be independent and identically log-normal distributed with parameters μ_1 and σ^2, i.e., $w_{1i} \sim \log N(\mu_1,\sigma^2), i = 1,\ldots,n$. Similarly, let $\tilde{w}_{1i}$ be independent and identically log-normal distributed with parameters μ_2 and σ^2, $\tilde{w}_{1i} \sim \log N(\mu_2,\sigma^2)$, $i = 1,\ldots,n$. Assume that w_{1i} and $\tilde{w}_{1j}$ are independent for $1 \leq i,j \leq n$. Define $w_{2i} = w_{1i}(\tilde{w}_{1i}+1)$, followed by $w_{2i} - w_{1i} = w_{1i}\tilde{w}_{1i}$. It can be shown that $w_{2i} - w_{1i} = w_{1i}\tilde{w}_{1i}$ and $\frac{w_{2i}-w_{1i}}{w_{2i}}$ are both log-normally distributed, particularly, $w_{2i} - w_{1i} \sim \log N(\mu_1 + \mu_2, 2\sigma^2)$ and $\frac{w_{2i}-w_{1i}}{w_{2i}} \sim \log N(\mu_2,\sigma^2)$. Define $X_i = \log(w_{2i} - w_{1i})$ and $Y_i = \log\left(\frac{w_{2i}-w_{1i}}{w_{1i}}\right)$. Then, both X_i and Y_i are normally distributed with $\mu_X = \mu_2 + \mu_1$ and $\mu_Y = \mu_2$.

Case 1: $H_0: \mu_X = \mu_0$ versus $H_a: \mu_X > \mu_0$

Consider the statistic $\hat{\mu}_X = \frac{1}{n}\sum_{i=1}^{n} \log(w_{2i} - w_{1i})$. Under the null hypothesis H_0, $\sqrt{\frac{n}{2}}\frac{\hat{\mu}_X - \mu_0}{\sigma} \sim N(0,1)$. The null hypothesis is then rejected at significance level α if $\sqrt{\frac{n}{2}}\frac{|\hat{\mu}_X - \mu_0|}{\sigma} > z_{\alpha/2}$. To achieve a power level of $(1-\beta)$, the required sample size is $n = \frac{2(z_{\alpha/2}+z_\beta)^2\sigma^2}{\delta^2}$, where $\delta = |\mu - \mu_0|$.

Case 2: $H_0: \mu_Y = \phi_0$ versus $H_a: \mu_Y > \phi_0$

Consider the statistic $\hat{\mu}_Y = \frac{1}{n}\sum_{i=1}^{n} \log(\frac{w_{2i}-w_{1i}}{w_{1i}})$. Under the null hypothesis H_0, $\sqrt{n}\frac{\hat{\mu}_Y - \phi_0}{\sigma} \sim N(0,1)$. The null hypothesis is rejected at significance level α if $\sqrt{n}\frac{|\hat{\mu}_Y - \phi_0|}{\sigma} > z_{\alpha/2}$. To achieve a power level of $(1-\beta)$, the required sample size is $n = \frac{(z_{\alpha/2}+z_\beta)^2\sigma^2}{\Delta^2}$, where $\Delta = |\phi - \phi_0|$.

Case 3: $H_0: p_X = \eta$ versus $H_a: p_X > \eta$

Consider the statistic $\hat{p}_X = \sum_{i=1}^{n} \frac{r_i}{n}$. Define $r_i = \begin{cases} 1 \text{ if } X_i = \log(w_{2i} - w_{1i}) \geq \delta \\ 0 \text{ otherwise} \end{cases}$

and $p_X = P(X_i \geq \delta) = \bar{\Phi}\left((\delta - \mu_X)/\sqrt{2\sigma^2}\right)$. Using similar arguments as in Cases 1 and 2, the required sample size to achieve a power level of $(1 - \beta)$ is given as $n = \frac{(z_\alpha + z_\beta)^2 p_X(1 - p_X)}{(p_X - \eta)^2}$.

Case 4: $H_0: p_Y = \eta$ versus $H_a: p_Y > \eta$

Consider the statistic $\hat{p}_Y = \sum_{i=1}^{n} \frac{r_i}{n}$. Define $r_i = \begin{cases} 1 \text{ if } Y_i = \log(\frac{w_{2i} - w_{1i}}{w_{1i}}) \geq \Delta \\ 0 \text{ otherwise} \end{cases}$ and

$p_Y = P(Y_i \geq \Delta) = \bar{\Phi}\left((\Delta - \mu_Y)/\sigma\right)$. Then, to achieve a power of $1 - \beta$, the required sample size is given as $n = \frac{(z_\alpha + z_\beta)^2 p_Y(1 - p_Y)}{(p_Y - \eta)^2}$.

References

Akaike, H. 1974 . A new look at statistical model identification. *IEEE Transactions on Automatic Control*, 19, 716–723.

Chang, M. 2007. *Adaptive Design Theory and Implementation Using SAS and R.* Chapman and Hall/CRC Press, Taylor & Francis, Boca Raton, FL.

Chen, J. and Chen, C. 2003. Microarray gene expression. In *Encyclopedia of Biopharmaceutical Statistics*, Chow, S.C. (Ed.), Marcel Dekker, Inc., New York, pp. 599–613.

Chow, S.C. 2007 . Statistics in translational medicine. Presented at Current Advances in Evaluation of Research & Development of Translational Medicine. National Health Research Institutes, Taipei, Taiwan, October 19, 2007.

Chow, S.C. and Chang, M. 2006 . *Adaptive Design Methods in Clinical Trials.* Chapman Hall/CRC Press, Taylor and Francis, Boca Raton, FL.

Chow, S.C., Chang, M., and Pong, A. 2005. Statistical consideration of adaptive methods in clinical development. *Journal of Biopharmaceutical Statistics*, 15, 575–591.

Chow, S.C. and Shao, J. 2006. On non-inferiority margin and statistical tests in active control trials. *Statistics in Medicine*, 25, in press.

Chow, S.C., Shao, J., and Hu, O.Y.P. 2002. Assessing sensitivity and similarity in bridging studies. *Journal of Biopharmaceutical Statistics*, 12, 385–400.

Efron, B. 1983. Estimating the error rate of a prediction rule: Improvement on cross-validation. *Journal of American Statistical Association*, 78, 316–331.

Efron, B. 1986. How biased is the apparent error rate of a prediction rule? *Journal of American Statistical Association*, 81, 461–470.

Gunst, G.F. and Mason, R.L. 1980. *Regression Analysis and Its Application*. Marcel Dekker, Inc., New York.

Hung, H.M.J. 2003. Statistical issues with design and analysis of bridging clinical trial. Presented at the 2003 Symposium on Statistical Methodology for Evaluation of Bridging Evidence, Taipei, Taiwan.

Hung, H.M.J., Wang, S.J., Tsong, Y., Lawrence, J., and O'Neil, R.T. 2003. Some fundamental issues with non-inferiority testing in active controlled trials. *Statistics in Medicine*, 22, 213–225.

ICH E5. 1998. International Conference on Harmonization Tripartite Guideline on Ethnic Factors in the Acceptability of Foreign Data. The U.S. Federal Register, Vol. 83, 31790–31796.

Johnson, N.L. and Kotz, S. 1970. *Distributions in Statistics—Continuous Univariate Distributions—1*. John Wiley & Sons, New York.

Li, L., Chow, S.C., and Smith, W. 2004. Cross-validation for linear model with unequal variances in genomic analysis. *Journal of Biopharmaceutical Statistics*, 14, 723–739.

Liu, J.P., Hsueh, H.M., and Hsiao, C.F. 2002. Bayesian approach to evaluation of the bridging studies. *Journal of Biopharmaceutical Statistics*, 12, 401–408.

Mallows, C.L. 1973. Some comments on Cp. *Techniometrics*, 15, 661–675.

Mankoff, S.P., Brander, C., Ferrone, S., and Marincola, F.M. 2004. Lost in translation: Obstacles to translational medicine. *Journal of Translational Medicine*, 2, 14.

Pizzo, P.A. 2006. *The Dean's Newsletter*. Stanford University School of Medicine, Stanford, California.

Rutgeerts, P., Sandborn, W.J., Feagan, B.G., Reinisch, W., Olson, A., Johanns, J., et al. 2005. Infliximab for induction and maintenance therapy for ulcerative colitis. *New England Journal of Medicine*, 353, 2462–2476.

Shao, J. 1993. Linear model selection by cross-validation. *Journal of American Statistical Association*, 88, 486–494.

Shao, J. and Chow, S.C. 2002. Reproducibility probability in clinical trials. *Statistics in Medicine*, 21, 1727–1742.

Shao, J. and Chow, S.C. 2007. Variable screening in predicting clinical outcome with high-dimensional microarrays. *Journal of Multivariate Analysis*, 98, 1529–1538.

Shibata, R. 1981. An optimal selection of regression variables. *Biometrika*, 68, 45–54.

Shih, W.J. 2001. Clinical trials for drug registrations in Asian Pacific countries: proposal for a new paradigm from a statistical perspective. *Controlled Clinical Trials*, 22, 357–366.

Tibshirani, R. 1996. Regression shrinkage and selection via the Lasso. *Journal of Royal Statistical Society B*, 58, 267–288.

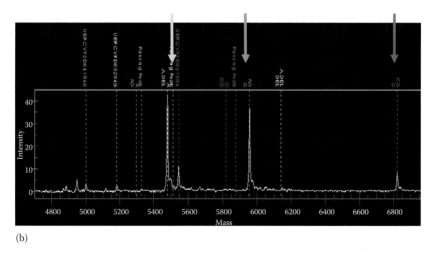

(b)

FIGURE 3.2: Analysis of polymorphisms using primer extension assays coupled with MALDI-TOF MS analysis.

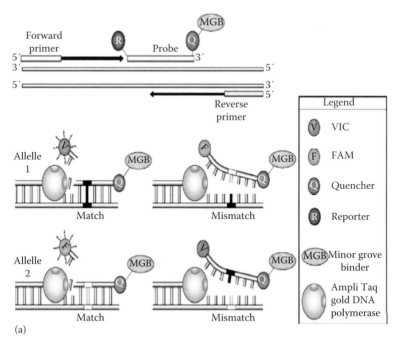

(a)

FIGURE 3.3: Taqman allelic discrimination. (a) Allelic discrimination using PCR amplification with two PCR primers.

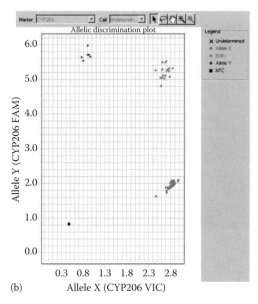

(b)

FIGURE 3.3: (continued) (b) Cluster plot showing fluorescence patterns for homozygote samples for Allele X (red) and Allele Y (blue), and XY heterozygotes (green).

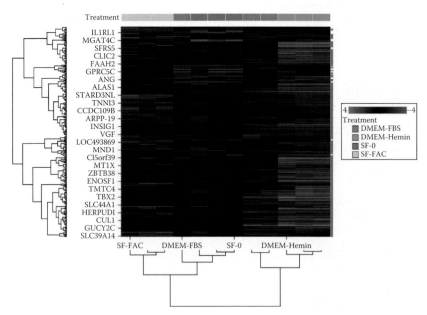

FIGURE A.3.6: Hierarchical clustering of significant genes.

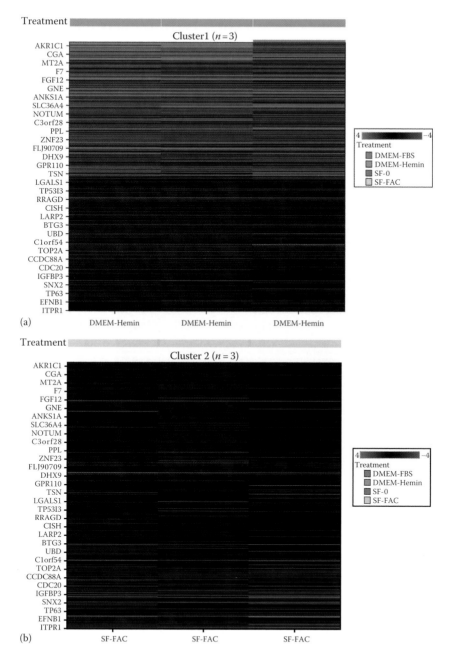

FIGURE A.3.7: (a) NMF, cluster 1, group 2, high iron (hemin), (b) NMF, cluster 2, group 4, normal iron (FAC).

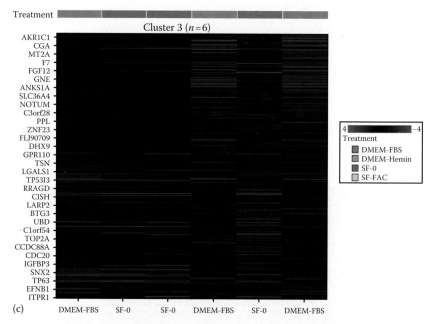

FIGURE A.3.7: (continued) (c) NMF, cluster 3, groups 1 and 3.

Chapter 7

Nonparametric Methods in Translational Research

Kongming Wang and Shein-Chung Chow

Contents

7.1 Introduction

Translational research translates the information from bench (e.g., basic research discoveries) to bedside (e.g., clinical application such as first-in-human). The translational process involves the investigation of the relations between the basic research discoveries and their clinical applications. In practice, these relatonships are often described by regression models. Given the complicated processes involved in the translational process, the regression models are more complicated than linear models. Statistical methods for linear/regression models are well established under certain distribution assumptions. However, these assumptions may not be bound in practice. As an alternative, it is suggested that nonparametric methods be considered. Nonparametric methods are useful without many assumptions, which can be applied regardless of the availability of analytical solutions (e.g., finite sample or asymptotic formula). With the massive computing power available, nonparametric methods are attractive in the case where analytical solutions do exist.

Once the model (relationship) between observations is obtained from bench (e.g., basic research discoveries) and bedside (e.g., clinic), it is of interest to evaluate the accuracy and reliability of the translational process. A typical approach is to assess the closeness between the observed values from bedside and the predicted values based on the observations obtained from bench under the established model. For this purpose, the following four criteria are commonly considered: (1) mean squared error of the absolute difference between the observed values and the predicted values, (2) mean squared error of the relative difference between the predicted values and the observed values, (3) the probability that the absolute difference between the predicted value and the observed value is within a prespecified small number, (4) the probability that the relative difference between the predicted value and the observed value is within a prespecified small number. In this chapter, we will focus on the criteria based on the relative difference between the predicted value and the observed value (i.e., points (2) and (4)).

Nonparametric methods are widely used in many different settings. To apply any of the four criteria, predicted values have to be computed. For this purpose, some local linear regression methods (kernel estimators, smoothing splines, local polynomials, linear wavelet shrinkage) for continuous response variable and local logit regression for binary response variable will be introduced. Bootstrap method will also be introduced for nonparametric estimation of standard errors of estimators such as the four criteria, confidence intervals for unknown parameters, and p-values for satistical testing. These methods will be applied in several cases. The first is validating parametric models. The idea is to test the equality of the predicted values from nonparametric regression and those from parametric modeling. The second is to compare regression functions such as responses of different treatment arms of a clinical trial. The responses can be estimated for each arm using nonparametric methods, and equality of the responses is then tested.

This chapter is organized as follows. In Section 7.2, the criteria (both local and global) for assessing the closeness between a predicted value and the observed value based on the mean squared error is introduced. Bootstrap is presented in Section 7.3 for assessing the accuracy of estimators or p-values for hypothesis testing. Section 7.4 provides nonparametric methods for local linear estimation. Our attention will be directed to cases where the response variable is binary in Section 7.5. Tests of parametric modeling and comparisons of regression curves are given in Sections 7.6 and 7.7, respectively. The application based on the probability that the relative difference between the predicted value and the observed value is within a prespecified small number is discussed in Section 7.8. A numerical example is given in Section 7.9 to illustrate the use of nonparametric methods described in this chapter. Section 7.10 provides brief concluding remarks.

7.2   Criterion Based on Mean Squared Error

Let (X,Y) be the pair of observations from basic research discoveries (e.g., pharmacokinetic data or gene expression) and clinical outcomes (e.g., toxicity, the presence of adverse events, or efficacy). An important question is the relationship between X and Y. A regression analysis is usually used to characterize the relationship between X and Y. In regression analysis, one wants to estimate Y by $g(X)$ for some function g after having observed X such that $g(X)$ is close to Y. If closeness means minimizing the mean squared error, then

$$E(g(X) - Y)^2 = \min_r E(r(X) - Y)^2.$$

Let $m(x) = E(Y|X = x)$ be the regression function. Then, m is the solution of the above minimization problem. Given a sample $(X_1, Y_1), \ldots, (X_n, Y_n)$ and unknown distribution of (X, Y), one needs to construct an estimate $m_n(x) = m_n(x, (X_1, Y_1), \ldots, (X_n, Y_n))$ of $m(x)$. Note that m is often nonlinear even in simple cases. By definition,

$$m(x) = \int y f(y|x) \, dy = \int y \frac{f(x,y)}{f(x)} \, dy,$$

where $f(y|x)$ is the conditional density of Y given $X = x$, $f(x,y)$ is the joint density of (X, Y), and $f(x)$ is the density of X. To simplify notation, we use f for all three densities. Assume that $f(x,y) = x + y$ for $0 \leq x, y \leq 1$ and $f(x,y) = 0$ otherwise. Then

$$m(x) = \frac{x + 2/3}{2x + 1}.$$

The accuracy of the translational process can be measured by local or global criteria based on mean squared error of the relative difference between the predicted values and the observed values. In other words, the local criterion is defined by the mean squared error of the relative difference between the estimator $m_n(x)$ and the unknown regression function $m(x)$ as follows:

$$l_n(x) = E[(m_n(x) - m(x))/m(x)]^2.$$

On the other hand, the global criterion is given by

$$L_n = E \int [(m_n(x) - m(x))/m(x)]^2 f(x) \, dx.$$

One may consider either local or global criterion based on the scope of the translational study, or both criteria if necessary.

Mean squared error of the absolute difference are similar and a bit simpler. Local criteria takes the form $E[(m_n(x) - m(x))]^2$ while global criteria takes the form $E \int [(m_n(x) - m(x))]^2 f(x) \, dx$.

As it can be seen, these criteria depend on the unknown functions $m(x)$ and $f(x)$. Thus, they cannot be applied directly. One way to deal with this problem is to derive the asymptotics of the criteria and substitute $m(x)$ and $f(x)$ with their estimates $\hat{m}(x)$ and $\hat{f}(x)$ in the asymptotic formula, respectively. Note that the Bootstrap method can also be used to estimate the distributions of $l_n(x)$ and L_n.

Translational study should be in both ways. One can formulate the regression problem from clinical observation to basic research as $r(y) = E(X|Y = y)$. Note that this formulation of the problem has a broad meaning if m is not monotonic. An example is that Y is a binary response variable and X takes more than two possible values (e.g., genotypes or a continuous variable). In such cases, $r(y)$ is a set of values instead of a single value. The local and global measurements $l_n(x)$ and L_n can be formally defined in terms of some metrics such as Lebegue measure if X has a continuous distribution. For more discussion on two-way translaton, see Chapter 3 of this book. By interchanging the role of X and Y, the nonparametric methods discussed in this chapter are applicable to obtain the closeness between the observed value X and the predicted value $\hat{r}(y)$. By bootstrapping the joint distribution of $(\hat{m}(x),\hat{r}(y))$, similar criteria for two-way translation can be defined as in Section 7.2.

If some a priori knowledge about the relationship between X and Y are known, then a parametric model such as a linear model or logistic regression can be assumed. Logistic regression has been used to model dose–response curve in humans based on priori knowledge from experiments in animals. Very often, one does not have enough a priori knowledge to make a good model assumption, and a mis-specified model could lead to false conclusions. Nonparametric methods do not rely on a priori knowledge other than very general assumptions (e.g., m and f are twice continuously differentiable), and nonparametric estimation is data-driven. The downside is that there are infinitely many parameters to be estimated. In practice, one has finite samples, sometimes a small sample. The asymptotic approximation to the finite sample distribution in such cases will be poor. Therefore, we will discuss bootstrap methods for estimating the distributions of the error measurements $l_n(x)$ and L_n.

7.3   Bootstrap

Bootstrap is a data-based simulation method for statistical inference. It can be used to find standard errors of estimators, confidence intervals for unknown parameters, and p-values for test statistics under a null hypothesis. Bootstrap is an attractive method owing to many factors such as small sample size, no analytic formula, too complicated even if analytic formula exists, massive computing power, and extensive research providing proper bootstrap procedure for an arbitrary statistical model.

Bootstrap can be described as a "plug-in" method (Boos, 2003). Given a sample $X_1,\ldots,X_n$, the interest is to estimate a functional of the underlining distribution F, which is a member of a set of distributions under a statistical model. For example, the mean is $T(F) = \int x dF(x)$ and the median is $Q(F) = F^{-1}(0.5)$. The bootstrap estimate of $T(F)$ and $Q(F)$ is $T(\hat{F})$ and $Q(\hat{F})$, respectively, where $\hat{F}$ is an estimate of F. For mean and median, the usual estimate is $T(F_n)$ and $Q(F_n)$, respectively, where F_n is the empirical distribution function.

The standard error of $T(F_n)$ can be estimated by using sample variance, and approximate confidence interval can be obtained by using percentiles of standard normal distribution. Such a "standard" estimate for standard error of $Q(F_n)$ does not exist if F is non-normal. We see how bootstrap can be employed to obtain estimated standard error of $Q(F_n)$. Draw random sample of size n with replacement from $X_1,\ldots,X_n$. Let $X_1^*,\ldots,X_n^*$ denote the sample and let F_n^* be the empirical distribution. Then, $Q(F_n^*)$ is a bootstrap estimate of the median. Repeating this resampling procedure B times, we have B bootstrap estimates of the median. The empirical distribution of these B median estimates is an approximation to the distribution of $Q(F_n)$ and the standard deviation of this empirical distribution is an estimate of the standard error of $Q(F_n)$. Bootstrap procedures with improved accuracy for constructing confidence intervals has been discussed in DiCiccio and Efron (1996).

As shown in the median case, the major step in bootstrapping is resampling. If the original samples $X_1, \ldots, X_n$ are i.i.d. and the goal is to estimate standard error or confidence interval of a functional $Q(F)$, then reampling can be randomly sampling with replacement as above. For finding p-value of a statistical test, resampling has to be restricted to satisfy the null hypothesis. Boos (2003) illustrated this point with the null hypothesis of equal mean H_0: $\mu_X = \mu_Y$. The test statistics is Welch's

$$t_w = (\bar{X} - \bar{Y}) / \sqrt{s_X^2/n + s_Y^2/m},$$

based on samples $X_1, \ldots, X_n$ and $Y_1, \ldots, Y_m$. To satisfy the null hypothesis of equal mean in the bootstrap world, a resampling procedure is to draw from $X_1 - \bar{X}, \ldots, X_n - \bar{X}$ and $Y_1 - \bar{Y}, \ldots, Y_m - \bar{Y}$, respectively. For nonparametric regression with heteroscedastic errors where the errors may be independent but not identically distributed, the wild bootstrap, which matches the moments of the observed error distribution around the estimated regression function at each design point, should be used (Brown and Heathcote, 2002). Resampling procedure such as block bootstrap (Politis and Romano, 1994), which draws blocks of consecutive observations with replacement to capture the dependence structure of neighbored observations, should be employed in case of dependent error.

A similar and handy method for error estimates in a statistic is jackknifing (Efron, 1979, 1982). The basic idea of jackknife and bootstrap are the same: estimating the variability of a statistic by the variability of the statistic between subsamples. Jackknife is less general than bootstrap but easier to implement. Chatterjee (1998) showed that jackknife schemes are special cases of generalized bootstrap. Jackknifing may result in slightly different results from bootstrapping. For example, to estimate standard error of a statistic, bootstrap will give slightly different results each time while jackknife will always give the same result if the number of leave-out observations is unchanged.

Note that software for bootstrap procedures are available online (e.g., www.insightful.com/downloads/libraries). SAS provides a macro jackboot.sas (http://support.sas.com /kb /24 /982.html) for bootstrapping and jackknifing. One could also write his/her own program in SAS for bootstrapping (Barker, 2005).

7.4 Local Linear Estimation

The commonly used methods (kernel estimators, smoothing splines, local polynomials, linear wavelet shrinkage) for estimating the regression function are linear methods in the sense that they are weighted averages of the observed responses

$$m_n(x) = \sum_{i=1}^{n} w_i(x|b, X_1, \ldots, X_n)Y_i, \tag{7.1}$$

where w_i are weights depending on design data points X_i, $i = 1,\ldots,n$, a smoothing parameter b (bandwidth) indicating the extent of smoothing, and the point x at which the function is being estimated. If $b \to 0$, then $w_i(x) \to 1$ if $x = X_i$ and is not defined elsewhere. In this case, the estimate m_n is an interpolation of the data with $m_n(X_i) = Y_i$. If $b \to \infty$ then $w_i(x) \to 1/n$ for all x and $m_n(x) \to \bar{Y} = \sum Y_i/n$. In this case, the estimate is a constant function (the sample mean of Y). Therefore, the bandwidth is crucial for these methods. A focal point in these methods is the selection of the smoothing parameter b. Many methods (global, local, data-driven) have been proposed for this purpose. The selection of b depends on the noise level and the smoothness of m and f.

Nadaraya (1964) and Watson (1964) proposed the weights

$$w_i(x|b,X_1,\ldots,X_n) = K\left(\frac{x-X_i}{b}\right) \Big/ \sum_{j=1}^{n} K\left(\frac{x-X_j}{b}\right),$$

where K is a kernel function, which is usually chosen to satisfy $K(x) = K(-x)$ and to have compact support. The Epanechnikov kernel

$$K(x) = 3/[4(1-x^2)_+], \quad x \in (0,1)$$

is optimal in the sense that it minimizes the mean square error (MSE), which is the sum of variance and square of the bias (Gasser et al., 1985). The estimator m_n is as smooth as the kernel function. So if m is twice continuously differentiable, then K has to be twice continuously differentiable. Under proper assumptions such as $\int |K(x)|dx < \infty$ and $\lim xK(x) = 0$ as $x \to \infty$, it is well known that $m_n(x) - m(x)$ has an asymptotically normal distribution (Jennen-Steinmetz and Gasser, 1988). The leading term of the asymptotic bias is $b^2 C_1(x)/2$ and the leading term of the asymptotic variance is $C_2(x)/(nb)$, where

$$C_1(x) = (m''(x) + 2m'(x)f'(x)/f(x))\mu_2(x)$$

and

$$C_2(x) = \sigma^2(x)V(K)/f(x).$$

Therefore, $(m_n(x) - m(x))/m(x)$ has an asymptotically normal distribution and

$$l_n(x) = \frac{b^4}{4}\left\{\frac{C_1(x)}{m(x)}\right\}^2 + \frac{1}{nb}\left\{\frac{C_2(x)}{m^2(x)}\right\} + o(1).$$

In the above formula, m' and m'' are the first- and second-order derivatives of m, respectively, and $\sigma^2(x) = \mathrm{Var}(Y|X = x)$. The two constants $\mu_2(K) = \int x^2 K(x)dx$ and $V(K) = \int K^2(x)dx$ depend on the kernel K only. The asymptotically optimal bandwidth that minimizes $l_n(x)$ is of the order $b = O(n^{1/5})$:

$$b_{\mathrm{opt}} = \left(\frac{C_2(x)}{nC_1^2(x)}\right)^{1/5}.$$

The error measurement $l_n(x)$ depends on the asymptotic mean, variance, and optimal bandwidth, which in turn depend on the unknown functions m, f, and their derivatives. One way to estimate the size of $l_n(x)$ is to estimate m, f, and their derivatives and ignore the higher order term $o(1)$. Many methods have been developed for estimating the optimal bandwidth.

The plug-in method uses an estimate of σ^2 and estimates of m, f, and their derivatives in the formula for b_{opt}. Gasser et al. (1986) proposed a simple estimator of σ^2. Derivatives of m can be estimated by kernel method similar to Equation 7.1 with a proper kernel K and bandwidth. The order of the bandwidth for estimating $m^{(k)}$ is $O(n^{-1/(2k+1)})$. For details, see Gasser and Muller (1984). These pilot estimates (optimal bandwidth, derivatives of m and f) can substitute for the unknown parameters in the bias and variance formula to get the approximate distribution of $(m_n(x) - m(x))/m(x)$. Confidence intervals and hypothesis testing can be carried out based on the approximate distribution.

Another handy method is cross-validation (Shao, 1993), which selects the bandwidth to minimize

$$\sum_{i=1}^{n} [(Y_i - \hat{m}_i(X_i))/\hat{m}_i(X_i)]^2,$$

where $\hat{m}_i(X_i)$ is the estimated response at X_i without using the data point (X_i, Y_i).

These bandwidth selection methods are adaptive to the data. The difficulty of the plug-in method lies in the estimation of the derivatives and small sample size. Very often, the sample size is limited, so the asymptotic distribution is a rough estimate of the finite sample distribution. The error of estimating derivatives is much larger than that of estimating m and f.

Another way of estimating the size of $l_n(x)$ is to bootstrap its distribution. Bootstrapping has been studied extensively for estimating the distributions of complicated statistics. For the nonparametric regression setting, it can be carried out as follows:

1. First select a bandwidth and get an estimate $\hat{m}$ of m. The bandwidth can be selected by plug-in method or cross-validation (Shao, 1993).

2. Compute the centered residuals

$$\hat{\varepsilon}_i = \eta_i - \frac{1}{n} \sum_{j=1}^{n} \eta_j,$$

where $\eta_i = Y_i - \hat{m}(X_i)$, $i = 1, \ldots, n$.

3. Resample with replacement from $\hat{\varepsilon}_i$. Denote the resampled residuals by ε_i^*, $i = 1, \ldots, n$. One can construct the resampled data as (X_i, Y_i^*) where $Y_i^* = \hat{m}(X_i) + \varepsilon_i^*$, $i = 1, \ldots, n$.

4. Smoother the resampled data in step (3) using the selected bandwidth in step (1) and denote the estimator by m^*. Now one can calculate an estimate $l^*(x)$ of the local error $l_n(x)$ using $(m^*, \hat{m})$ instead of (m_n, m).

Repeat steps (3) and (4) N times, then the distribution of the $\{l_j^*(x),\ j = 1,\ldots,N\}$, is a good estimate of the distribution of $l_n(x)$.

Similarly, the distribution of L_n can be estimated by bootstrapping the estimated residuals. The only change from the above steps is in step (4), where an estimate L^* of L_n is calculated instead of $l^*(x)$. One can derive the asymptotic leading term of L_n and use pilot estimates of σ and the derivatives of m and f. But the formula is a bit complicated and the asymptotic approximation is not good if sample size is small.

Other popular linear methods include smoothing splines and local polynomial fitting. The local polynomial estimator $\hat{m}(x)$ is obtained by locally weighted polynomial regression to minimize the weighted sum of squared residuals

$$\min_{a(x),b_1(x),\ldots,b_k(x)} \sum_{i=1}^{n} K((x-X_i)/b)[Y_i - a(x) - b_1(x)(x-X_i) - \cdots - b_k(x)(x-X_i)^k]^2.$$

As in kernel regression, K is a kernel and b a smoothing parameter. This leads to the estimator $\hat{m}(x) = a(x)$. Local linear fit ($k = 1$) has been used most frequently. With $k = 0$ (local constant fitting), the resulted estimator is the Nadaraya–Watson kernel estimator. With $k = 1$, the properties of the estimator are similar to that of Nadaraya–Watson kernel estimator: the asymptotic variance is the same as the asymptotic variance for $k = 0$ while the asymptotic bias does not have the term involving m' and f'. It, therefore, needs no pilot estimators for m' and f' to apply the plug-in method.

A smoothing spline is the solution to the penalized regression problem $\min_m S_b(m)$ where

$$S_b(m) = \sum_{i=1}^{n} (Y_i - m(X_i))^2 + b \int (m''(x))^2 dx.$$

Here, b is a roughness penalty parameter analogous to the bandwidth of the kernel estimator. For a given smoothing parameter $0 < b < \infty$, the resulting estimator $\hat{m}$ is a natural cubic spline (piecewise cubic polynomial with continuous second-order derivative) with knots at X_i, $i = 1,\ldots,n$ (Reinsch, 1967). One of the often used methods for calculating smoothing splines is to use a set of basis functions known as B-splines, which are defined by the recurrence formula (DeBoor, 1978). Silverman (1984) presented smoothing spline as a kernel estimator asymptotically. Hence, the asymptotic properties of smoothing spline is similar to that of kernel estimator.

The techniques (plug-in, cross-validation, bootstrapping) discussed for kernel estimators can be applied to local polynomial fitting and smoothing splines (Fan and Gijbels, 1995, Gu, 1998; Seifert and Gasser, 2006). For example, bandwidth selection by cross-validation for local polynomial fitting is to minimize

$$\sum_{i=1}^{n} [(Y_i - \hat{m}_i(X_i))/\hat{m}_i(X_i)]^2,$$

where $\hat{m}_i(X_i)$ is the estimated response at X_i by local polynomial fitting without using the data point (X_i, Y_i).

7.5 Binary Response

If Y is a binary response variable (e.g., $Y = 1$ for responder and $Y = 0$ for nonresponder), the regression problem becomes

$$p(x) = Pr(Y = 1 | X = x). \tag{7.2}$$

The Nadaraya–Watson estimator is then a weighted proportion

$$p_n(x) = \sum_{i:Y_i=1} w_i(x|b,X_1,\ldots,X_n).$$

When X takes finite values (e.g., disease stages or genotypes), the data can be organized as (X_i, Y_{ij}) for $i = 1,\ldots,I$ and $j = 1,\ldots,n_i$, where X_i, $i = 1,\ldots,I$, are distinctive values of X, and there are n_i subjects with covariate value X_i. Let $Y_{i\cdot} = \sum_{j=1}^{n_i} Y_{ij}$. Then, $Y_{i\cdot}$ has a binomial distribution binomial$(n_i, p(X_i))$. The Nadaraya–Watson estimator based on data $(X_i, Y_{i\cdot})$ is given by

$$\hat{p}_n(x) = \sum_{i=1}^{I} w_i(x|b,X_1,\ldots,X_n)Y_{i\cdot} \Bigg/ \sum_{i=1}^{I} w_i(x|b,X_1,\ldots,X_n)n_i.$$

Let $\bar{Y}_i = Y_{i\cdot}/n_i$. Then, the Nadaraya–Watson estimator based on data $(X_i, \bar{Y}_i)$ has the form

$$\bar{p}_n(x) = \sum_{i=1}^{I} w_i(x|b, X_1,\ldots,X_n)\bar{Y}_i \Bigg/ \sum_{i=1}^{I} w_i(x|b, X_1,\ldots,X_n).$$

Local polynomial fitting and smoothing splines could be modified to estimate $p(x)$ (e.g., restricting the estimators in $[0, 1]$), but it may result in nondifferentiable estimators. Instead of local polynomial fitting, other local models such as local logit model is more appropriate. For local logit model,

$$p(x) = E(Y|X = x) = \frac{1}{1 + e^{-x\theta_x}}.$$

Then, the estimate of $p(x)$ is given by (Gozalo and Linton, 2000)

$$\hat{p}(x) = E(Y|X = x) = \frac{1}{1 + e^{-x\hat{\theta}_x}},$$

where $\hat{\theta}_x$ is the solution of the following minimization problem

$$\min_{\theta_x} \sum_{i=1}^{n} K((x - X_i)/b)(Y_i - \frac{1}{1 + e^{-X_i\theta_x}})^2.$$

Bandwidth b can be selected by cross-validation. Simulation of Frolich (2006) shows that local logit regression has better finite sample performance than the Nadaraya–Watson estimator or local linear fitting.

7.6   Testing Parametric Model

Parametric models are frequently used to describe the association between a response variable and its predictors. Linear model $m(x) = E(Y|X = x) = \alpha + \beta x$ is a good example. The adequacy of such parametric models often needs to be validated. Conventional methods check if there are any trends in the residuals. If a trend is smaller than the noise level, it cannot be accurately detected. Even if a trend is observed, adjustment to the parametric model is still not easy.

Nonparametric methods can be applied to check/validate parametric models and provide hints for model adjustment if the parametric model does not fit the data well. Assume a parametric model $g(x,\theta)$ for the regression function m. One wants to test

$$H_0: m(x) = g(x,\theta_0), \quad \text{all } x$$

versus   (7.3)

$$H_1: m(x) \neq g(x,\theta_0), \quad \text{for some } x$$

for a known function g and unknown parameter θ_0. For continuous m and g, the alternative hypothesis H_1 means that m and g differ in a set of positive size (e.g., positive Lebesgue measure). Let $\hat{\theta}$ be an estimate of θ_0 based on a given data set (X_i,Y_i), $i = 1,\ldots,n$. The parameter θ can be estimated by least-square fit or maximum likelihood estimate (MLE). The least-square fit $\hat{\theta}$ is the solution of the minimization problem

$$\min_{\theta} \sum_{i=1}^{n} (Y_i - g(X_i,\theta))^2.$$

Let $m_n(x)$ be a nonparametric estimate of m. Then, the following statistics:

$$D_n = \sum_{i=1}^{n} (m_n(X_i) - g(X_i,\hat{\theta}))^2$$

can be used to test the hypothesis H_0. If H_0 is not rejected, then the parameter model $g(x,\theta_0) = E(Y|X = x)$ is validated. We will assume $\hat{\theta} - \theta_0 = O(n^{-1/2})$. In many cases, such as estimator exists (e.g., least-square estimator in a linear model).

To derive the critical values for the statistic D_n at a given significance level, we need to know the finite sample distributions of these statistics. For linear model $g(x,\theta) = u'(x)\theta$ where $\theta = (\alpha,\beta)'$ and $u(x) = (1,x)'$, the least-square estimate is $\hat{\theta} = P_n Y$ where $P_n = (U_n U_n')^{-1} U_n'$ is a $2 \times n$ matrix, with $Y = (Y_1,\ldots,Y_n)'$ and $U_n = (u(X_1),\ldots,u(X_n))$. Similarly, a linear nonparametric estimate as discussed in Section 7.4 can be written as $m_n(x) = W_n'(x)Y$ where

$$W_n(x) = (w_1(x|b,X_1,\ldots,X_n),\ldots,w_n(x|b,X_1,\ldots,X_n))'.$$

Now

$$m_n(X_i) - g(X_i,\hat{\theta}) = W_n'(X_i)Y - u'(X_i)P_n Y,$$

and

$$D_n = Y'ZZ'Y,$$

where

$$Z' = \begin{pmatrix} W_n'(X_1) - u'(X_1)P_n \\ \vdots \\ W_n'(X_n) - u'(X_n)P_n \end{pmatrix}.$$

If the conditional distribution of $Y|X$ is mutltinomial, then $D_n|X$ has a noncentral Chi-square distribution with degree of freedom of rank(ZZ'). So the critical value for testing H_0 versus H_1 can be calculated or looked up from the available tables.

For complicated parametric model $g(x,\theta)$, the exact distribution of D_n is not easy to derive. As discussed above, two methods can be applied to estimate the distribution of D_n: the "plug-in" method based on asymptotics and the bootstrap method. Earbark et al. (2005) derived the asymptotics of D_n by calculating the leading term of its bias and variance. Then

$$(D_n - \text{bias})/\sqrt{\text{variance}}$$

has a normal distribution asymptotically. The bias and variance most likely depend on the unknown parameter θ_0 and the smoothing parameter, so that both can be estimated and then "pluged-in" to the bias and variance formula. With complicated bias and variance formula and limited data, this plug-in method may not work well. The following is an algorithm for bootstrapping the distribution of D_n (Brown and Heathcote, 2002).

Let $\tilde{\varepsilon}_i = Y_i - g(X_i,\hat{\theta})$ be the residuals of the parametric regression. Center the residuals $\tilde{\varepsilon}_i$ from the assumed model

$$\bar{\varepsilon}_i = \tilde{\varepsilon}_i - \frac{1}{n}\sum_{j=1}^{n} \tilde{\varepsilon}_j.$$

If data are generated from the assumed model $Y_i = g(X_i,\theta_0) + \varepsilon_i$ and ε_i are iid random variables with mean 0, then $\bar{\varepsilon}_i$ are almost iid distributed with mean 0. The bootstrap procedure is the following:

1. Draw n numbers ε_i^* from $\{\bar{\varepsilon}_i\}$ with replacement and form the bootstrapped data as

$$Y_i^* = g(X_i,\hat{\theta}) + \varepsilon_i^*.$$

2. Use the same nonparametric procedure and same bandwidth that resulted in m_n to get an estimate m_n^* of the regression function m, using data (X_i,Y_i^*), $i = 1,\ldots,n$.

3. Compute

$$D_n^* = \sum_{i=1}^{n} (m_n^*(X_i) - g(X_i,\hat{\theta}))^2.$$

Repeat steps (1)–(3) B times (say $B = 1000$). Then, the empirical distribution of $\{D_n^*\}$ is an approximation of the distribution of D_n under the hypothesis H_0. Given a significance level, H_0 can be tested by comparing the percentiles of $\{D_n^*\}$ and D_n.

If the error terms ε_i are nonstationary (e.g., $\varepsilon_i = \varepsilon_i(X_i)$), then wild bootstrap, which matches the moments of the observed error distribution around the estimated regression function at each design point, should be used.

7.7   Comparison of Regression Curves

In randomized clinical trials, one is interested in comparing two regression curves. For example, if Y denotes the treatment effect, then two regression curves $m_1(x)$ and $m_2(x)$ represent the expected value of Y under treatment and control, respectively, given some covariates $X = x$ (e.g., baseline prognostic factors). If $m_1(x) = m_2(x)$ for all x, there will be no treatment difference between the two groups while $m_1 \geq m_2$ but $m_1 \neq m_2$ indicates an improved efficacy under treatment. One might want to test

$$H_0: m_1 = m_2 \quad \text{versus} \quad H_1: m_1 \neq m_2 \tag{7.4}$$

given data (X_{1i}, Y_{1i}), $i = 1, \ldots, n_1$, and (X_{2j}, Y_{2j}), $j = 1, \ldots, n_2$.

Let $\hat{m}_1$ and $\hat{m}_2$ be nonparametric estimates of m_1 and m_2, respectively. The local linear estimators discussed in Section 7.4 could be employed to get $\hat{m}_1$ and $\hat{m}_2$. We will assume that the distributions of X_1 and X_2 have the same support. This is the case for randomized clinical trials where subjects are assigned to treatment and control groups randomly. Many trials use stratified randomization to balance important covariates. If X_1 and X_2 have disjoint support, then the information about the regression functions m_1 and m_2 are obtained in disjoint regions and it is difficult to compare the two regression functions.

Srihera and Stute proposed an intuitive two-sample score test statistic for testing the hypothesis H_0. The test statistic takes the form

$$\hat{T} = \frac{1}{n_1 n_2} \sum_{i=1}^{n_1} \sum_{j=1}^{n_2} W\left(\frac{X_{1i} + X_{2j}}{2}\right) \left[\hat{m}_1\left(\frac{X_{1i} + X_{2j}}{2}\right) - \hat{m}_2\left(\frac{X_{1i} + X_{2j}}{2}\right)\right].$$

This is the average of the weighted difference between $\hat{m}_1$ and $\hat{m}_2$ at $n_1 n_2$ points. Under some technical assumptions, it was shown that under H_0,

$$\frac{\sqrt{N}\hat{T}}{\hat{\sigma}} \xrightarrow{L} N(0,1),$$

where

$$N = n_1 n_2 / (n_1 + n_2)$$

is the standardized factor for $\hat{T}$ in terms of n_1 and n_2, $\hat{\sigma}$ is a consistent estimator of the conditional variance of Y_{11} given X_{11}, and $\xrightarrow{L}$ denotes convergence in distribution.

They also show that $\sqrt{N}\hat{T}$ is asymptotically normal under alternative hypothesis H_1. Based on the asymptotics under H_1, the weight function W can be chosen to maximize the ratio of (asymptotic mean)^2/(asymptotic variance) of $\sqrt{N}\hat{T}$. They presented a W that maximizes the power of the test when the two regression functions differ by a multiple of a fixed function.

Munk and Dette (1998) rewrite the test problem as

$$H_0 : M^2 = 0 \quad \text{versus} \quad H_1 : M^2 \neq 0$$

and proposed an estimate of M^2 directly from the data, where M^2 is the L^2 norm of $m_1 - m_2$. Let $\{X_{1,(i)}\}$ be the order statistics of $\{X_{1i}\}$ and let $Y_{1,(i)}$ denote the corresponding response of $X_{1,(i)}$. Let $Y_{1,(0)} = Y_{1,(1)}$ and $Y_{1,(n_1+1)} = Y_{1,(n_1)}$, and similarly define $\{Y_{2,(j)}\}$. The estimator is

$$\hat{M}^2 = \sum_{i=0}^{n_1} \sum_{j=0}^{n_2} \lambda_{ij}(Y_{1,(i+1)} - Y_{2,(j+1)})(Y_{1,(i)} - Y_{2,(j)}),$$

where the weights are given by

$$\lambda_{ij} = (X_{1,(i+1)} \wedge X_{2,(j+1)} - X_{1,(i)} \vee X_{2,(j)}) I_{\{X_{1,(i+1)} \wedge X_{2,(j+1)} > X_{1,(i)} \vee X_{2,(j)}\}}.$$

The notations $a \wedge b = \max\{a,b\}$ and $a \vee b = \min\{a,b\}$ are used. Under some conditions, it is shown that

$$\sqrt{n_1 + n_2}(\hat{M}^2 - M^2)$$

is asymptotically normal with mean 0. The asymptotic variance is a complex function of the unknown regression functions m_1 and m_2 as well as the unknown variance functions of the regression model.

These test statistics are intutively defined and can be computed from data. The problem is to estimate the standard error of these statistics so that the hypothesis testing could be carried out. Asymptotic formula is complicated and requires estimates of unknown functions. Bootstrap method can be applied to estimate the standard error of the test statistics, similar to testing a parametric model. Assuming $E(\varepsilon_{ij}) = 0$ and $V(\varepsilon_{ij}) = \sigma_i^2$, $i = 1,2$. Note that the variances may be unequal ($\sigma_1^2 \neq \sigma_2^2$) in the regression models.

First estimate the centered residuals by

$$\hat{\varepsilon}_{ij} = Y_{ij} - \hat{m}_i(X_{ij}) - \sum_{j=1}^{n_i}[Y_{ij} - \hat{m}_i(X_{ij})]/n_i,$$

$j = 1,\ldots,n_i$ and $i = 1,2$, where $\hat{m}_i$ is a nonparametric estimate of m_i. We will consider the kernel estimates

$$\hat{m}_i(x) = \sum_{j=1}^{n_i} w_i(x|b_i, X_{i1}, \ldots, X_{in_i})Y_{ij},$$

where $i = 1,2$.

Draw random samples of size n_i from $\{\hat{\varepsilon}_{ij}, j = 1,\ldots,n_i\}$, $i = 1,2$, respectively. Denote these resamples by $\{\hat{\varepsilon}_{ij}^*, j = 1,\ldots,n_i\}$, $i = 1,2$ and calculate the bootstrap data as

$$Y_{ij}^* = \hat{m}_1(X_{ij}) + \hat{\varepsilon}_{ij}^*.$$

Note that the two regression functions are identical for the bootstrap data. This is required under the null hypothesis. This also requires the estimate of m_1 at $\{X_{2j}, j = 1,\ldots,n_2\}$.

Now compute the test statistic from the bootstrap data Y_{ij}^*. Suppose we want to use the test statistic $\hat{T}$. It is the same procedure if the test statistic $\hat{M}^2$ is used. To compute the test statistic $\hat{T}^*$ based on the bootstrap sample, the two regression functions have to be estimated from the bootstrap data using the same nonparametric method. If a smoothing technique as described in Section 7.4 is used, the same smoothing parameters for computing $\hat{T}$ should be used to compute $\hat{T}^*$.

Repeat the above bootstrap procedure B times and denote the bootstrap statistic by $\{\hat{T}_j^*, j = 1,\ldots,B\}$. The empirical distribution of $\{\hat{T}_j^*, j = 1,\ldots,B\}$ is an approximation to the distribution of $\hat{T}$ under the null hypothesis. A p-value for testing the null hypothesis can be obtained by $p = (B^* + 1)/(B + 1)$ where B^* is the number of bootstrap repeats with $\hat{T}_j^* \geq \hat{T}$.

7.8 Probability-Based Criterion

Discussions in the previous sections used moment-based criteria. Probability-based local criterion is now

$$p(x,\delta) = P\{|l_n(x)| < \delta\} = P\{|(m_n(x) - m(x))/m(x)| < \delta\}$$

or

$$p(x,\delta) = P\{|m_n(x) - m(x)| < \delta|m(x)|\}.$$

This criteria is based on the relative difference of observed and predicted values. The criteria based on absolute difference takes the form $P\{|m_n(x) - m(x)| < \delta\}$.

For the local linear estimators discussed in Section 7.4, the estimator $m_n(x)$ is a weighted average of the observations. The theory of large deviations applies to this weighted average. Joutard (2006) derived sharp large deviations for the Nadaraya–Watson estimator under some proper assumptions. Let $f(x,y)$ be the joint density function of (X,Y) and let $f_1'(x,y)$ be the derivative of f with respect to the first variable. For $\alpha > 0$, define two entropy functions

$$I_{m,\alpha}(t) = \int_{R^2} [\exp(t(y - m(x) - \alpha)K(u)) - 1] f(x,y) \mathrm{d}u \mathrm{d}y$$

and

$$J_{m,\alpha}(t) = \int_{R^2} u[\exp(t(y - m(x) - \alpha)K(u)) - 1] f_1'(x,y) \mathrm{d}u \mathrm{d}y,$$

where K is the kernel function. Choose bandwidth b such that $\lim_{n\to\infty} nb = \infty$ and $\lim_{n\to\infty} nb^2 = c \geq 0$. Then for large n,

$$P(m_n(x) - m(x) > \alpha) = \frac{\exp[nbI_{m,\alpha}(\tau) + cH_{m,\alpha}(\tau)]}{\tau(2\pi nbI''_{m,\alpha}(\tau))^{1/2}}(1 + o(1)),$$

where τ is such that $I'_{m,\alpha}(\tau) = 0$ and $H_{m,\alpha}(t) = -(I^2_{m,\alpha}(t)/2 + J_{m,\alpha}(t))$. Similarly,

$$P(m_n(x) - m(x) < -\alpha) = \frac{\exp[nbI_{m,-\alpha}(-\tau) + cH_{m,-\alpha}(-\tau)]}{\tau(2\pi nbI''_{m,-\alpha}(-\tau))^{1/2}}(1 + o(1)),$$

where τ is such that $I'_{m-\alpha}(-\tau) = 0$. Replacing α by $\delta|m(x)|$, one has an explicit formula for the asymptotics of the probability-based local criteria $P\{|l_n(x)| < \delta\}$.

The asymptotics depend on the unknown functions $m(x)$ and $f(x,y)$ and bandwidth b. These functions can be estimated by the methods of Section 7.4. The bandwidth can be selected by plug-in method or cross-validation. These estimates can be substituted into the above formula to calculate the probability-based local criteria $P(|l_n(x)| < \delta)$ by dropping the $o(1)$ term. The formula is rather complicated and the large deviation boundaries are valid only for a large sample size.

To avoid the complexity, one can employ bootstrap to get an estimate of the distribution of $l_n(x)$ as described in Section 7.4. Let $\{l^*_k(x), k = 1, \ldots, B\}$ be the bootstrap estimates of the local criteria $l_n(x)$ in B replications as in Section 7.4. The probability-based local criteria can be computed from the bootstrap distribution as follows. For a given δ, let

$$B_\delta = \sum_{j=1}^{B} r^*_j,$$

where $r^*_j = 1$ if $|l^*_j(x)| < \delta$ and $r^*_j = 0$ otherwise. Then, $p^*(x,\delta) = B_\delta/B$ is the bootstrap estimate of $p(x,\delta) = P(|l_n(x)| < \delta)$.

Hypothesis testing problems such as

$$h_0 : p(x,\delta) < p_0 \quad \text{versus} \quad h_1 : p(x,\delta) \geq p_0$$

can also be carried out based on the bootstrapped estimates of $l_n(x)$, where p_0 and δ are prespecified values. Note that the bootstrap estimates are independent replications. Therefore B_δ has a binomial distribution in the bootstrap world. The p-value for testing the hypothesis h_0 versus h_1 (one-tailed test) can be calculated by

$$p = P(Y \geq B_\delta),$$

where Y has a binomial distribution binomial(B, p_0). If this p-value is smaller than the prespecified significance level (usually 0.05), then hypothesis h_0 is rejected and h_1 is accepted.

7.9   Numerical Example

Kernel smoothing and parametric model validation are performed in this section using simulated data. Program is in S/SPlus language. Data are generated with the model

$$y_i = m(x_i) + \sigma\varepsilon_i, \quad x_i = 0.01i, \quad i = 1,\ldots,100, \tag{7.5}$$

where $m(x) = 20x + 3\sin(10x)$. One can think of the covariate x as a normalized gene expression and the response y as the clinical outcome (e.g., survival time, percentage of tumor shrinkage) after treatment with an experimental medicine in translational research. The goal is to find the relationship between baseline gene expression and the clinical outcome. Nonparametric regression will be used to estimate the relationship, and bootstrap technique will be used to test parametric models for the relationship. Two parametric models will be tested:

M1:	$m(x\|\alpha,\beta) = \alpha + \beta x$
M2:	$m(x\|\alpha,\beta,\delta,\eta) = \alpha + \beta x + \delta\sin(\eta x)$

where M1 is a linear model and M2 is the correct model.

7.9.1   Nonparametric Regression

For a specified σ, data (x_i, y_i), $i = 1,\ldots,100$, are generated by the above model. Kernel smoothing, with "normal" kernel as in SPlus and the optimal bandwidth b_{opt} selected by cross-validation to minimize the sum of squared errors

$$\sum_{i=1}^{100}(\hat{m}_b^i(x_i) - y_i)^2,$$

is employed to estimate the regression function nonparametrically. Here, $\hat{m}_b^i$ is the kernal estimate of m with bandwidth b and without using data point (x_i, y_i).

The true optimal bandwidth b_{true} is obtained by a grid search to minimize the true sum of squared errors

$$\sum_{i=1}^{100}(\hat{m}_b(x_i) - m(x_i))^2,$$

where $\hat{m}_b$ is the kernel estimate of m with bandwidth b and the "normal" kernel.

Simulations with 10 different σ and 20 replications for each σ show that, on average, bandwidth selected by cross-validation is close to the true optimal bandwidth for all levels of σ (Table 7.1). Kernel estimate of the regression function is plotted in Figure 7.1.

7.9.2   Validating Parametric Model

To validate a specified parametric model, the parameters of the parametric model have to be estimated from the data. Model M1 is a linear model and parameters

TABLE 7.1: Results with 20 simulated data sets.

σ	SNR	Mean (b_{true})	Mean (b_{opt})	Reject M1	Reject M2
1	19.4	0.08	0.09	19	0
2	9.70	0.12	0.13	20	0
3	6.47	0.14	0.16	19	0
4	4.85	0.16	0.18	18	0
5	3.88	0.19	0.19	11	0
6	3.23	0.22	0.23	5	0
7	2.77	0.23	0.21	6	0
8	2.43	0.26	0.28	3	0
9	2.16	0.29	0.29	2	0
10	1.94	0.30	0.29	4	0

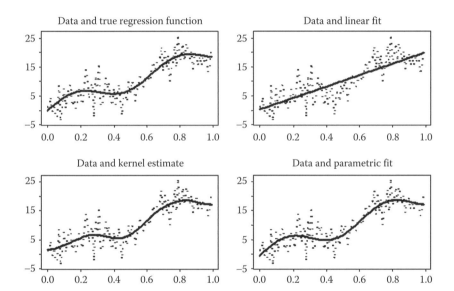

FIGURE 7.1: A typical run with $\sigma = 4$.

are estimated by linear regression. Model M2 is a nonlinear model and parameters are chosen to minimize the sum of squared errors $\sum(y_i - m(x_i|\alpha,\beta,\delta,\eta))^2$ using the SPlus function "nlmin." Let $\hat{m}_K$ be the nonparametric estimation of the regression function by kernel smoothing, let $\hat{m}_L$ be the linearly fitted function (model M1), and let $\hat{m}_N$ be the nonlinearly fitted function (model M2). The difference between the nonparametric estimation and the parametric estimations can be calculated by

$$d_L = \sum_{j=1}^{100} [\hat{m}_K(x_j) - \hat{m}_L(x_j)]^2,$$

$$d_N = \sum_{j=1}^{100} [\hat{m}_K(x_j) - \hat{m}_N(x_j)]^2.$$

To test model M1, the bootstrap data are generated by

$$y_i^* = \hat{m}_L(x_i) + \varepsilon_i^*, \quad i = 1, \ldots, 100,$$

where $\{\varepsilon_i^*\}$ are randomly resampled residuals with replacement from the centered residuals

$$\hat{\varepsilon}_i = y_i - \hat{m}_L(x_i) - \frac{1}{100} \sum_{j=1}^{100} [y_j - \hat{m}_L(x_j)], \quad i = 1, \ldots, 100.$$

The bootstrapped data (x_i, y_i^*) are smoothed by kernel smoothing using the "normal" kernel and the optimal bandwidth b_{opt}. Denote the smoothed function by $\hat{m}_K^*$. The difference between $\hat{m}_K^*$ and $\hat{m}_L$ is

$$d_L^* = \sum_{j=1}^{100} [\hat{m}_K^*(x_j) - \hat{m}_L(x_j)]^2.$$

Repeat the bootstrap procedure 1000 times, the bootstrap p-value for testing the null hypothesis $\{H_0:$ model M1 is true$\}$ is calculated as

$$p = \frac{\{\text{number of bootstrap replications with } d_L^* > d_L\} + 1}{1000 + 1}.$$

If p is smaller than a prespecified significance level (usually 0.05), then H_0 is rejected.

The procedure for testing model M2 is the same as that for testing model M1. The only difference is to use $\hat{m}_N$ and d_N instead of $\hat{m}_L$ and d_L.

A typical run with $\sigma = 4$ resulted in $b_{\text{opt}} = 0.21$ and bootstrapped p-values of 0.008 for testing model M1 and of 0.984 for testing model M2. Model M1 is rejected, meaning that data are not generated from a linear model, while model M2 is accepted. Data and estimated functions are plotted in Figure 7.1.

The simulation is carried out for 10 different σ. For each σ, 20 sets of data are generated and the above procedure is run for each set of data. Simulation results are summarized in Table 7.1. The columns of Table 7.1 are σ, signal to noise ratio SNR $= \max |f(x)|/\sigma$, average of the 20 true optimal bandwidths, average of the 20 optimal bandwidths selected by cross-validation, number of runs with model M1 rejected, and number of runs with model M2 rejected.

Bandwidth selected by cross-validation increases as SNR decreases. This is expected because larger bandwidth should be used if data present higher noise level. The bootstrap procedure rejects incorrect model M1 in at least 90% of the 20 runs if SNR ≥ 4.85, and it never rejects the correct model M2. A model is rejected if the bootstrap p-value is less than 0.05.

This small simulation suggests that the nonparametric methods are applicable to translational research. Technology has been advanced to obtain genome data with improved SNR, e.g., SNR $= 9$ (Mein et al., 2000) and SNR $= 10$ (Hesse et al., 2006). Similarly, SNR of medical images could be higher than 20 (Huang et al., 2008). With SNR ≥ 9, the simulation shows that the wrong model is rejected with high probability (at least 95% of the simulations).

7.10   Concluding Remarks

Bootstrap is very attractive if analytic solutions are complicated or if there is no analytic solution. The crucial step in a Bootstrap procedure is resampling. While non-restricted bootstrap procedures can be used to estimate standard errors of statistics and confidence intervals of parameters, restricted Bootstrap, which forces resampling under the null hypothesis, should be used to compute p-values for hypothesis testing. As Bootstrap software is developing, its use is becoming more widespread.

The local linear estimators of regression functions and the test statistics for validating parametric models or for testing the equality of two regression functions can all be extended to cases with a high-dimensional predictor. The extension is straightforward. The problem in high dimensions is the sparsity of data. Ideas such as additive model, where the regression function takes the form $m(x_1, \ldots, x_p) = \sum m_j(x_j)$, have been proposed and developed. In practice, regression functions with two-dimensional predictor (e.g., images) are most often encountered and sparsity is usually not a big problem.

The methods can also be extended to semiparametric models $m(x,z) = \alpha + \beta z + m_0(x)$ where z are some covariates such as age and gender. If α and β are known, then $m_0(x) = m(x,z) - (\alpha + \beta z)$ is a nonparametric regression function. On the other hand, if m_0 is given, then $m(x,z) - m_0(x) = \alpha + \beta z$ is a linear model. So, an iterative algorithm can be used to estimate (α, β) and m_0 alternatively until convergence. Hypothesis testing procedures as described in the previous sections can be applied to semiparametric models.

Finally, nonparametric methods are well known for survival analysis (Bewick et al., 2004; Akritas, 2004). The Kaplan–Meier method for estimating survival curves, the log-rank test for comparing survival curves of two treatment groups, and the Cox regression for estimating hazard ratio and effects of explanatory variables are all well received by the pharmaceutical industry and the regulatory agencies around the globe. SAS has procedures to perform these analyses (proc lifetest, proc phreg).

References

Akritas, M. 2004. Nonparametric survival analysis. *Stat. Sci.*, 19, 615–623.

Barker, N. 2005. A practical introduction to the Bootstrap using the SAS system. www.lexjansen.com/phuse/2005/pk/pk02.pdf.

Bewick, V., Cheek, L., and Ball, J. 2004. Statistics review 12: Survival analysis. *Crit. Care*, 8, 389–394.

Boos, D. 2003. Introduction to the Bootstrap world. *Stat. Sci.*, 18, 168–174.

Brown, S. and Heathcote, A. 2002. On the use of nonparametric regression in assessing parametric regression models. *J. Math. Psych.*, 46, 716–730.

Chatterjee, S. 1998. Another look at the jackknife : Further examples of generalized bootstrap. *Stat. Probab. Lett.*, 40, 307–319.

DeBoor, C. 1978. *A Practical Guide to Splines*. New York: Springer-Verlag.

DiCiccio, T. and Efron, B. 1996. Bootstrap confidence intervals. *Stat. Sci.*, 11, 189–228.

Efron, B. 1979. Bootstrap methods: Another look at the jackknife. *Ann. Stat.*, 7, 1–26.

Efron, B. 1982. The jackknife, the bootstrap, and other resampling plans. *In Society of Industrial and Applied Mathematics CBMS-NSF Monographs*, 38.

Fan, J. and Gijbels, I. 1995. Data-driven bandwidth selection in local polynomial fitting: Variable bandwidth and spatial adaptation. *J. R. Stat. Soc. Ser. B*, 57, 371–394.

Frolich, M. 2006. Non-parametric regression for binary dependent variables. *Econometrics Journal*, 9, 511–540.

Hesse, J., Jacak, J., Kasper, M., Regl, G., Eichberger, T., Winklmayr, M., Aberger, F., Sonnleitner, M., Schlapak, R., Howorka, S., Muresan, L., Frischauf, A., and Schutz, G. 2006. RNA expression profiling at the single molecule level. *Genome Res.*, 16, 1041–1045.

Huang, S., Vader, D., Wang, Z., Stemmer-Rachamimov, A., Weitz, D., Dai, G., Rosen, B., and Deisboeck, T. 2008. Using magnetic resonance microscopy to study the growth dynamics of a glioma spheroid in collagen I: A case study. *BMC Med. Imaging*, 8(3), doi:10.1186/1471-2342-8-3.

Gasser, T. and Müller, H. 1984. Estimating regression functions and their derivatives by the kernel method. *Scan. J. Stat.*, 11, 171–185.

Gasser, T., Müller, H., and Mammitzsch, V. 1985. Kernels for nonparametric curve estimation. *J. R. Stat. Soc. Ser, B*, 47, 238–252.

Gasser, T., Sroka, L., and Jennen-Steinmetz, C. 1986. Residual variance and residual pattern in nonlinear regression. *Biometrika*, 73, 625–633.

Gozalo, P. and Linton, O. 2000. Local nonlinear least square: Using parametric information in nonparametric regression. *Journal of Economics*, 99, 63–106.

Gu, C. 1998. Model indexing and smoothing parameter selection in nonparametric function estimation. *Statistica Sinica*, 8, 607–646.

Jennen-Steinmetz, C. and Gasser, T. 1988. A unifying approach to nonparametric regression estimation. *JASA*, 83, 1084–1089.

Joutard, J. 2006. Sharp large deviations in nonparametric estimation. *Nonparam. Stat.*, 18, 293–306.

Mein, C., Barratt, B., Dunn, M., Siegmund, T., Smith, A., Esposito, L., Nutland, S., Stevens, H., Wilson, A., Phillips, M., Jarvis, N., Law, S., de Arruda, M., and Todd, J. 2000. Evaluation of single nucleotide polymorphism typing with invader on PCR amplicons and its automation. *Genome Res.*, 10(3), 330–343.

Munk, A. and Dette, H. 1998. Nonparametric comparison of several regression functions: Exact and asymptotic theory. *Ann. Stat.*, 26, 2339–2368.

Nadaraya, E. 1964. On estimating regression. *Th. Prob. Appl.*, 9, 141–142.

Politis, D. and Romano, F. 1994. The stationary bootstrap. *J. Am. Stat. Assoc.*, 89, 1303–1313.

Reinsch, C. 1967. Smoothing by spline functions. *Numerische Mathematik*, 10, 177–83.

Serfert, B. and Gasser, T. 2006. Local polynomial smoothing. *In Encyclopedia of Statistical Sciences*, John Wiley & Sons, Inc.

Shao, J. 1993. Linear model selection by cross-validation. *J. Am. Stat. Ass.*, 88, 486–494.

Silverman, B. 1984. Spline smoothing: The equivalent variable kernel method. *Ann. Stat.*, 12, 898–916.

Srihera, R. and Stute, W. Nonparametric comparison of regression functions. http://centrumjh.karlin.mff.cuni.cz/SEMINAR/Stute.pdf

Watson, G. 1964. Smooth regression analysis. *Sankhya*, A, 26, 359–372.

Chapter 8

Model Selection/Validation*

Jen-pei Liu

Contents

8.1 Introduction

Molecular and heritable targets of many diseases can be identified after completion of the Human Genome Project (HGP) (Casciano and Woodcock, 2006; Dalton and Friend, 2006; Varmus, 2006). For example, imatinib mesylate is targeted at the BCR-ABL protein tyrosine kinase resulting from a reciprocal translocation between the long arms of chromosomes 9 and 22 in the patients who suffer from chronic myeloid leukemia (CML). On the other hand, both trastuzumab and lapatinib are selected inhibitors for the encoded protein of human epidermal growth-factor receptor (HER2), which is over-expressed and amplified in 20%–30% of the patients with metastatic breast cancer. These are the two examples for which a particular molecular target has been identified and an agent is developed for that specific target. However, other genome-wide approaches have been employed to select treatment regimens based on the prognosis or prediction of the clinical outcomes from the gene-expression profiles of a set of genes. For example, Oncotype DX breast-cancer assay employs the technical platform of reverse-transcriptase-polymerase chain reaction (RT-PCR) to measure the expression levels of 21 genes for prognosis of tumor

---

* Disclaimer: The views expressed in this chapter are personal opinions of the authors and may not necessarily represent the outlook of National Taiwan University, Taipei, Taiwan and the National Health Research Institutes, Zhunan, Taiwan.

recurrence in patients with breast cancer receiving hormonal therapy (Paik et al., 2004, 2006). Currently, the United States National Cancer Institute (NCI) is conducting the TAILORx (Trial Assigning Individualized Options for Treatment) trial, in which the patients with a recurrence score of 11–25 as determined by Oncotype DX breast-cancer assay are randomly assigned to receive either adjuvant chemotherapy plus hormonal therapy or adjuvant hormonal therapy alone (Sprarano et al., 2006). On the other hand, the MINDACT (Microarray in Node-negative Disease may Avoid ChemoTherapy) trial sponsored by the European Organization for Research and Treatment of Cancer (EORTC) randomizes patients with early-stage breast cancer with a high-risk clinical prognosis and a low-risk molecular prognosis of distant metastasis, based on a 70-gene microarray, MammaPrint, to the use of either clinico-pathologic criteria or gene signature in treatment decisions for the possible avoidance of chemotherapy (MINDACT, 2006; van't Veer et al., 2002; Van de Vijver et al., 2002). These trials are examples of translational research, which have an important implication for the future individualized treatments for thousands of breast-cancer patients (Swain, 2006). In addition, both Oncotype DX breast-cancer assay and the MammaPrint are based on multiple heritable markers and, hence, are classified as a new class of In Vitro Diagnostic Multivariate Index Assays (IVDMIAs).

A testing device for the identification of the molecular or heritable targets is used for all the above-mentioned trials. Owing to the importance and consequence of the diagnostic results, which predict response to the treatment of trastuzumab, the devices for identification of over-expression of HER2 protein or amplification of *HER2* gene are designated as Class III devices, which require clinical trials by the premarket application (PMA). On the other hand, the MammaPrint is only for breast-cancer prognosis, and is not intended for diagnosis, prediction, or detection of responses to therapy or to help select the optimal therapy (Decision Summary k0762694; FDA, 2007e). It is designated as a Class II device under regulation 510(k) of premarket notification. Other characteristics of the diagnostic devices for the molecular targets are that they are heritable markers or multiple markers investigated simultaneously (multiplex tests). Success of translational medicine (TM) depends on the accuracy and quality of the assays for the molecular targets. To meet the different requirements of sensitivity, specificity, and quality for validation of diagnostic devices used in the TM and targeted clinical trials, the U.S. Food and Drug Administration (FDA) recently issued several important guidances or draft guidance. These guidances include

Guidance on *Gene Expression Profiling Test System for Breast Cancer Prognosis* (May 9, 2007; FDA, 2007a).

Guidance on *Pharmacogenetic Tests and Genetic Tests for Heritable Markers* (June 19, 2007; FDA, 2007b).

Draft Guidance on *In Vitro Diagnostic Multivariate Index Assays* (July 26, 2007; FDA, 2007c).

Statistical Guidance on Reporting Results from Studies Evaluating Diagnosis Tests (March 13, 2007; FDA, 2007d).

In addition, the *Journal of Biopharmaceutical Statistics* published a special issue on the medical device clinical studies, which addresses some issues and challenges of *in vitro* IVDMIA and DNA microarray studies. Furthermore, examples validation of assays for identification of over-expression/amplification of HER2 protein/gene and development of MammaPrint are given in the next section. Statistical considerations on model selection and validation for the devices of heritable markers are provided in Section 8.3, while discussion and final remarks are presented in the last section.

8.2 Examples

8.2.1 Assays for Identification of Over-Expression or Amplification of *HER2* Gene

As mentioned earlier, trastuzumab is indicated for

1. Adjuvant treatment for patients with *HER2*-over-expressing, node-negative breast cancer

2. Treatment of patients with metastasis breast cancer whose tumors over-express the HER2 protein and who have received one or more chemotherapy regimens for their metastatic disease

3. Combination therapy with paclitaxel for the treatment of patients with metastatic breast cancer, whose tumors over-express the HER2 protein and who have not received chemotherapy for their metastatic disease

Therefore, to receive any form of treatment of trastuzumab, *HER2* gene must be over-expressed or amplified in the patients with breast cancer. In the 2006 draft package inclusion of trastuzumab, there are two approved methods for HER2 detection. The first method is to measure the magnitude of over-expression of *HER2* gene by the immunohistochemistry (IHC) procedure. The other approach is to identify the amplification of *HER2* gene by fluorescent in situ hybridization (FISH) approach. Although different platforms are used for the identification of either over-expression of HER2 protein or amplification of *HER2* gene, the principles for ensuring the accuracy of the assays and quality control of the devices remain the same. These devices are indicated as an aid in the assessment of breast-cancer patients for whom trastuzumab therapy is being considered. Patients falsely identified as positive may be unnecessarily considered for receiving the treatment of trastuzumab. Consequently, she may be exposed to the avoidable risks of some potential serious adverse events, such as infusion toxicity or cardiotoxicity, or in some rare cases, death. On the other hand, patients falsely tested as negative will not receive the potential clinical benefit of the treatment with trastuzumab and may show very poor outcome, or even death. Therefore, the devices for HER2 detection are associated with the determination of use of a certain treatment and its potential clinical benefit and risk. Consequently, in addition to preclinical evaluation, the devices for detection of over-expression of HER2 protein or amplification of *HER2* gene are classified as Class III devices, which require clinical studies under the regulations of PMA.

BioGenex InSite Her-2/neu Mouse Monoclonal Antibody (Clone CB11) detection system is one of the devices recently approved by the U.S. FDA for the detection of over-expression of HER2 protein (FDA, 2004). It is intended for in vitro diagnosis of the IHC assays to semiquantitatively localize the over-expression of Her-2/neu in formalin-fixed, paraffin-embedded normal and neoplastic tissue sections, by light microscopy. InSite Her-2/neu is indicated as an aid in the assessment of breast-cancer patients for whom trastuzumab therapy is considered. To assure the quality of the product, preclinical tests of BioGenex InSite Her-2/neu consists of analytical specificity/cross-reactivity, stability, a number of different types of reproducibility studies as well as characterization of control cell lines. Reproducibility is one of the most important evaluations of the precision of the assay. In addition, as mentioned earlier, BioGenex InSite Her-2/neu is a semiquantitative assay with the following ordinal categorical scoring system from 0 to 3+:

- 0 (negative): no staining or membrane staining in <10% of tumor cells

- 1+ (negative): faint, barely perceptible membrane staining in >10% of tumor cells, where the cells are stained only in part of the membrane

- 2+ (positive): weak to moderate complete membrane staining observed in >10% of tumor cells

- 3+ (positive): strong, complete membrane staining in >10% of tumor cells

Therefore, the evaluation of reproducibility studies based on ordinal categorical data is different from the traditional methods using the continuous data (Chow and Liu, 1995). The following reproducibility studies were performed for BioGenex InSite Her-2/neu:

1. Intra-run reproducibility

2. Inter-run reproducibility

3. Manual versus automatic reproducibility

4. Detection systems reproducibility

5. Lot-to-lot reproducibility of the complete kit

6. Inter-laboratory reproducibility

The intra-run reproducibility study consisted of five different formalin-fixed, paraffin-embedded breast-cancer tissues with a range from 0 to 3+ for the semiquantitative immunostaining intensity score and one positive quality-control slide of 3+. Each specimen was run in a blinded randomized manner against one slide with the negative reagent control. The results of intra-run reproducibility study are given in Table 8.1. The agreement of results from the three slides in a single run is 100%. Therefore, this study shows that the intra-run reproducibility of BioGenex InSite Her-2/neu is adequate. The inter-run reproducibility study used the same positive quality-control slides and five breast-cancer tissue sections. However, the study was performed on three separate days with the same lot of BioGenex InSite Her-2/neu antibody and the same lot of detection reagents. The results of the inter-run reproducibility study are provided in Table 8.2. It can be observed from Table 8.2

TABLE 8.1: Summary of staining intensities of BioGenex InSite Her-2/neu on breast tissue sections obtained in a single run.

	First Slide		Second Slide		Third Slide	
	Her-2/neu[a]	NC[b]	Her-2/neu[a]	NC[b]	Her-2/neu[a]	NC[b]
Quality-control slides	3+	0	N/A	N/A	N/A	N/A
S98-388	0	0	0	0	0	0
S97-3352A	1+	0	1+	0	1+	0
S97-229	1+ ∼ 2+	0	1+ ∼ 2+	0	1+ ∼ 2+	0
S97-1324A	2+	0	2+	0	2+	0
S97-2357B	3+	0	3+	0	3+	0

Source: Approved summary of BioGenex InSite Her-2/neu (P040030).
[a] BioGenex InSite Her-2/neu.
[b] NC, negative control.

that the inconsistent results occur in three breast-cancer tissue sections. For tissue section S97-3352A, the first and third runs had an intensity score of $0 \sim 1+$, but second run produced a score of 0. For tissue section S97-229, both the first and second run yielded a score of $1+ \sim 2+$, but the third run gave a score of $1+$. Finally, for tissue section S97-1324A, both the second and third run showed an intensity score of $2+$, but for the first run, the score was $2+ \sim 3+$. Since, the test result is considered positive if it is at least $2+$, thus, inconsistent and compromised result occurred only in specimen S97-1324A. However, low reproducibility in the range from $1+$ to $2+$ by IHC should be reevaluated by another technical platform, such as FISH assay or by other evaluators.

TABLE 8.2: Summary of staining intensities of BioGenex InSite Her-2/neu on breast tissue sections obtained in three separate runs.

	First Run (Day1)		Second Run (Day 2)		Third Run (Day 3)	
	Her-2/neu[a]	NC[b]	Her-2/neu[a]	NC[b]	Her-2/neu[a]	NC[b]
Quality-control slides	3+	0	3+	0	3+	0
S98-388	0	0	0	0	0	0
S97-3352A	0 ∼ 1+	0	0	0	0 ∼ 1+	0
S97-229	1+ ∼ 2+	0	1+ ∼ 2+	0	1+	0
S97-1324A	2+ ∼ 3+	0	2+	0	2+	0
S97-2357B	3+	0	3+	0	3+	0

Source: Approved summary of BioGenex InSite Her-2/neu (P040030).
[a] BioGenex InSite Her-2/neu.
[b] NC, negative control.

TABLE 8.3:   Summary of staining intensities of BioGenex InSite Her-2/neu on breast tissue sections obtained in a manual versus automated system.

	Manual		Automated[a]	
	Her-2/neu[b]	NC[c]	Her-2/neu[b]	NC[c]
Quality-control slides	3+	0	3+	0
S98-388	0	0	0	0
S97-3352A	0	0	0	0
S97-229	1+	0	1+ ~ 2+	0
S97-1324A	2+	0	2+	0
S97-2357B	3+	0	3+	0

Source: Approved summary of BioGenex InSite Her-2/neu (P040030).
[a]   Performed on a BioGenex *i*6000 automated staining system.
[b]   BioGenex InSite Her-2/neu.
[c]   NC, negative control.

For the reproducibility comparing the manual method with the automated method, a single breast-cancer section from each of the same five breast-cancer tumor-tissue blocks was employed. Table 8.3 presents the results. The only inconsistent result occurred in S97-229 for which the manual method yielded a score of 1+ and the automated method provided a score of 1+ ~ 2+. However, this inconsistent result of S97-229 may yield different positive or negative diagnoses and require reevaluations. Three detection systems with different chromogens were used for the reproducibility, such that DAB (used in final Her-2/neu test kit) and AEC employed horseradish peroxidase, and Fast Red used alkaline phosphatase. The results are provided in Table 8.4. The variation between different chromogens seems much larger than that observed from the intra-run and between-run precision studies, and manual versus

TABLE 8.4:   Summary of staining intensities of BioGenex InSite Her-2/neu on breast tissue sections visualized by three different chromogens.

	DAB		AEC		Fast Red	
	Her-2/neu[a]	NC[b]	Her-2/neu[a]	NC[b]	Her-2/neu[a]	NC[b]
Quality-control slides	3+	0	N/A	N/A	N/A	N/A
S98-388	0	0	0 ~ 1+	0	0	0
S97-3352A	0	0	0 ~ 1+	0	0 ~ 1+	0
S97-229	1+	0	1	0	0 ~ 1+	0
S97-1324A	2+	0	2	0	1+ ~ 2+	0
S97-2357B	3+	0	3	0	3	0

Source: Approved summary of BioGenex InSite Her-2/neu (P040030).
[a]   BioGenex InSite Her-2/neu monoclonal antibody.
[b]   NC, negative control.

TABLE 8.5: Summary of inter-laboratory concordance of BioGenex InSite Her-2/neu.

| | | Labs | | |
	A	B	C	Counts
Results	−	−	−	5
	−	−	+	1
	−	+	−	2
	−	+	+	1
	+	+	−	2
	+	+	+	19
			Total	30

Source: Approved summary of BioGenex InSite Her-2/neu (P040030).

automated methods. Specimen S97-1324A yielded inconsistent semiquantitative immunostaining intensity scores of 2+, 2, and 1+ ∼ 2+ across Super Sensitive Detection Systems using DAB, AEC, and Fast Red, respectively. The phenomenon was observed between a scoring range of 1+ ∼ 2+. The inter-laboratory reproducibility study was conducted in all different, geographically distinct laboratories. The investigators followed the same manual IHC-staining protocol described in the package insert of BioGenex InSite Her-2/neu test kit and were provided the same 30 tissue blocks. These tissue blocks included 10 each of 3+ and 2+ Her-2/neu staining scores, and 5 each of 1+ and 0 Her-2/neu staining scores. A summary of the results of inter-laboratory concordance is given in Table 8.5. Labs A and B agreed on 27 blocks out of 30, resulting in a concordance rate of 90%. On the other hand, Labs A and C agreed on 26 blocks out of 30 with a concordance rate of 86%. It follows that the concordance rate between Labs B and C was 83% (25/30). Variability among the different laboratories was in the range from 10% to 17%. In summary, it can concluded that the reproducibility of BioGenex InSite Her-2/neu test kit is at least 80%, with inconsistency occurring mostly in the range from 1+ to 2+, which distinguishes a negative result from a positive finding. The seriousness of inconsistency between 1+ and 2+ depends on the prevalence of patients actually with the staining intensity scores 1+ and 2+.

One clinical study was conducted in a single-blind fashion with a total of 352 identical pairs of formalin-fixed, paraffin-embedded slides of anonymized breast-tumor specimen tissue sections to demonstrate the agreement between BioGenex InSite Her-2/neu test kit and the reference assay, the DakoCytomation HercepTest (P980018). An equal representation of positive and negative specimens was made. The objective of the clinical study was to prove that the percent agreement between the two detection systems is >75% with the following hypothesis:

$$H_o: P \leq 75\% \quad \text{versus} \quad H_a: P > 75\%,$$

where P is the percent agreement.

TABLE 8.6: 3×3 Concordance table from clinical study.

	HercepTest			
InSite Her-2/neu	$-$	2+	3+	Total
$-$	128	5	2	135
2+	25	80	9	114
3+	11	14	78	103
Total	164	99	89	352

Source: Approved summary of BioGenex InSite Her-2/neu (P040030).

The results of the clinical studies are summarized in Table 8.6, which is a 3×3 concordance table with grouping staining scores of 0 and 1 into one category of the negative finding. As shown Table 8.3, the overall percent agreement between the two detection systems is 81.3% (286/352) with a 95% confidence interval from 76.8% to 85.2%. Since, the lower limit of the 95% confidence interval is >75%, we can conclude that at 2.5% level, the percent agreement is >75%. In addition, the estimate of the κ-measure of agreement is 0.714 with a 95% confidence interval from 0.653 to 0.776. On the other hand, the percent positive agreement is 80.8% (80/99) with a 95% confidence interval from 71.7% to 88.8%. The percent positive agreement with respect to the cutoff of 3+ by HercepTest is 87.6% (78/89) with a 95% confidence interval from 79.0% to 93.7%. Percent negative agreement is 78.0% with a 95% confidence interval from 70.9% to 84.1%. Although the overall percent agreement is >75%, the percent positive agreement with respect to the threshold of 2+ by HercepTest and percent negative agreement of BioGenex InSite Her-2/neu test kit cannot be concluded to be >75% at the 2.5% significance level. If the staining scores of 2+ and 3+ were grouped into one category of the positive finding for a 2×2 concordance table, the overall percent was 87.8% (309/352) with a 95% confidence interval from 83.9% to 91.0%. Therefore, the same conclusion can be reached. However, the percent negative agreement of BioGenex InSite Her-2/neu test kit cannot be concluded to be >75%, as the lower limit of a 95% confidence interval was 70.9. As a result, up to 22% of inconsistent findings were found in this clinical study. It should be noted that as there is no gold standard, an agreeable result does not imply that the findings are correct.

8.2.2 MammaPrint

MammaPrint is a qualitative array-based *in vitro* device that uses the expression profile of a panel of 70 selected genes to assess a patient's risk for distant metastasis. It is one of the few prognostic devices based on the latest microarray technology approved by the U.S. FDA (FDA, 2007e). It is indicated for use by physicians as a prognostic marker only, along with other clinicopathological factors. However, it is not indicated for diagnosis, or to predict or detect response to therapy or help select the optimal therapy for patients. As a result, MammaPrint was classified as a Class II device under the regulation 510(K) of premarket notification.

The MammaPrint analysis is designed to determine the gene activity of specific genes in a tissue sample compared with a reference standard. The MammaPrint analysis produces the MammaPrint Index, which is the correlation of the gene-expression profile of the test sample with a template comprising the mean expression profile of 44 tumors with a good clinical outcome. The range of the MammaPrint Index is from -1 to $+1$ and the threshold is $+0.4$. If the MammaPrint Index of the tumor sample is $>+0.4$, then the patient is classified as having low risk for distant metastasis. If it is $\leq +0.4$, then the risk of distant metastasis for the patient is high. If the MammaPrint Index is in the borderline zone between 0.365 and 0.435, then the sample needs to be retested. The average MammaPrint Index is computed from the two test results. The sample will be reported as a borderline sample if the average MammaPrint Index is between 0.3775 and 0.4225. Since it is a pharmacogenetic test based on multiple heritable markers, the development of the test and evaluations for quality control and performance of the device is more complicated than that with a single marker.

Microarray is a one of the most important breakthrough technologies in the last decade. It allows one to investigate cancer biology by simultaneously examining the complete expression patterns of thousands of genes or an entire genome. In a subset of breast-cancer patients defined by age of 55 years or younger, tumor size <5 cm, no node involvement, and only receiving the local-regional treatment, van't Veer et al. (2002) observed that the expression profile of 231 genes was statistically significantly correlated with the occurrence of distant metastasis within 5 years. Subsequently, the profile from a subset of 70 genes from the original 231 was chosen to correlate with distant metastasis (Van de Vijver et al., 2002). However, this 70-gene signature was generated on microarrays consisting of about 25,000 60-mer oligonucleotides. Therefore, it is infeasible and costly to use these arrays in a high-throughput processing of large amount of samples for routine diagnostic practice. To overcome these shortcomings of the original arrays, MammaPrint adopted a new technology of miniarrays with eight identical subarrays of 1900 60-mer oligonucleotides per glass slide, which can be individually hybridized. About 232 reporter genes are printed in triplicate per subarray, including the 70 genes that make up the MammaPrint expression profile. In addition, each subarray contains 915 normalization genes and 289 spots for hybridization and printing quality control. As a result, besides the selection of genes, the validation of the MammaPrint includes the equivalence in the analytical performance between the MammaPrint and its original 25 k arrays, and clinical utility in the prognosis of distant metastasis over the current standard clinicopathological criteria.

Glas et al. (2006) reported the results of converting the original 25 k microarray to a miniarray for a routine diagnostic device. The original 78 tumor samples for the development of the original 25 k microarray were again used for the evaluation of the new 1900-feature miniarray. The Pearson correlation coefficient using the MammaPrint Indices of 78 samples between the original 25 k microarray and the 1900-feature miniarray was 0.924 with a *p*-value <0.0001. On the other hand, using a threshold of +0.4, seven discordant predictions were found between the original array and the miniarray. The percent agreement was 91.03% with a 95% confidence interval from 84.65% to 97.85%. As a result, at the 0.025 significance level, the percent agreement of the MammaPrint with the original 25 k array was > 80%. About 49 samples were amplified and hybridized for the second time on the same day, and the intra-class correlation coefficient was observed to be 0.995. This represents the intra-run technical reproducibility. To investigate whether the MammaPrint Index changes over time, a sample with low risk and another with high risk were tested repeatedly over a 100 times during a period of 12 months. The standard deviations of repeated measurements of MammaPrint Index did not exceed 0.028. A sample with the MammaPrint Index close to the threshold of +0.4 was analyzed 40 times. The misclassification rate for this sample was found to be 15% (6/40). This misclassification rate was close to that predicted under a normal distribution using the sample average of 0.430 and sample standard deviation of 0.028 from the 40 repeated measurements of MammaPrint Index. Although a CV of 6.5% seems rather low and acceptable, the misclassification rate could be lower if the technical variation can be further reduced.

Buyse et al. (2006) reported the results of clinical utility for the MammaPrint from a multinational collaborative initiative sponsored by the TRANSBIG consortium. The patient eligible criteria are (a) age <61 years old at diagnosis, (b) diagnosed before 1999 with node negative, (c) tumor size <5 cm, and (d) no prior adjuvant chemotherapy. Out of the 403 eligible patients, 302 had complete data. Unadjusted and adjusted hazard ratios were employed as criteria for clinical validation. The primary endpoints include the time to distant metastasis (TTDM), overall survival (OS), and disease-free survival (DFS). The sample size of 100 patients was determined to detect a hazard ratio of at least 2 with a 90% power at the 0.05 significance level for a two-sided test. The unadjusted hazard ratios were 2.32, 2.79, and 1.50 for TTDM, OS, and DFS, respectively. The hazard ratios adjusted for the clinical risk groups based on 10-year survival probability were 2.13, 2.63, and 1.36 for TTDM, OS, and DFS, respectively. Except for the adjusted hazard ratio for DFS at 10 years, all hazard ratios were statistically significant at the 0.05 level. The virtually unchanged magnitudes of the adjusted hazard ratios indicate that MammaPrint provides additional independent prognostic information over the clinicopathological criteria.

The overall accuracy for prognosis of distant metastasis can be evaluated by the area under the receiver's operating characteristic (ROC) curves. The areas of ROC curves for TTDM at 5 years and OS at 10 years were 0.681 and 0.648, respectively, by MammaPrint. On the other hand, the areas of ROC curves for TTDM at 5 years and OS at 10 years using adjuvant score based on the patient's age, tumor size and grade, ER status, and node involvement (Ravdin et al., 2001) were 0.659 and 0.576, respectively. Therefore, an increase of 2.2% and 7.2% in the prognostic accuracy for TTDM at 5 years and OS at 10 years were provided by MammaPrint. It is not known whether the differences in the area under ROC curves between MammaPrint and adjuvant score are statistically significant. In addition, the shapes and patterns of the ROC curves are strikingly different between MammaPrint and the adjuvant score. The additional classification accuracy provided by the MammaPrint does not occur until the false-positive rate reaches 0.3. When the false-positive rate is <0.3, the ROC curve of MammaPrint coincides with the $45°$ line. In other words, when the false-positive rate is restricted under 0.3, the prognostic accuracy of MammaPrint is no better than flopping of a fair coin. However, Buyse et al. (2006) argued that all available classification systems for patients with early-stage breast cancer try to identify reliably those patients with low risk of metastasis or death, even at the expense of high false-positive rate. Therefore, to compare the classification accuracy for the low risk of distant metastasis or death, instead of the overall area of ROC curve, the paired partial areas under the ROC curves between the MammaPrint and adjuvant score should be employed as the endpoint (Li et al., 2008).

8.3 Statistical Considerations

From the examples of the MammaPrint, it is very important to identify the genes with an expression profile that not only discriminates the patients with low risk from those with high risk, but also accurately predicts the future clinical outcome of a patient. In addition, selection of differentially expressed genes is a multistep tedious process. For example, initially a subset of 231 genes was identified using 25 k microarrays. Subsequently, a core of 70 genes was selected for the device product using the 1900-feature miniarray for the assessment of the risk of distant metastasis for patients with early-stage breast cancer. As the selection process involves tens of thousands of genes, control of falsely identified genes turns out to be a very critical and difficult task. Once the genes are chosen, the representation of the expression profile and determination of thresholds for classification of the diseased patients and nondiseased subjects subsequently become very important endeavors. On the other hand, although the principles for the quality control and analytical performance of the pharmacogenetic tests using heritable markers are identical, these devices derived from the latest technological breakthroughs require some special statistical considerations.

8.3.1 Selection of Genes and Representation of Expression Levels

Currently, the most widely available statistical methods for the identification of differentially expressed genes are based on the traditional hypotheses, testing for equality:

$$H_0: \mu_{Ti} - \mu_{Ci} = 0 \quad \text{versus} \quad H_a: \mu_{Ti} - \mu_{Ci} \neq 0, \tag{8.1}$$

where and μ_{Ti} and μ_{Ci} are the true average expression levels on the log-scale (base 2) of the gene i under the test condition (e.g., high risk) and the control condition (e.g., low risk), respectively, G is the total number of genes under investigation, $i = 1,...,G$ (Dudoit et al., 2002; Simon et al., 2003; Tusher et al., 2001; Wang and Ethier, 2004).

However, the traditional hypotheses testing for equality is only to detect whether the difference in the average expression levels between the test and control conditions is 0. It fails to take the magnitudes of the biologically meaningful fold changes into consideration. In addition, simultaneously testing tens of thousands of genes may render an extremely false-positive rate. Therefore, various multiple comparison procedures are applied to resolve this issue (Benjamini and Hochberg, 1995 Hochberg and Tamhane, 1987;). However, all these methods fail to take into account both the magnitudes of biologically meaningful fold change and the statistical significance at the same time. Since the goal is to select differentially expressed genes, the hypothesis for identification of differentially expressed genes should be formulated as the alternative hypothesis. On the other hand, gene i is said to be differentially expressed if the difference in the average expression levels between the tested and controlled conditions is either greater than a minimal biologically meaningful limit C_i (for over-expression) or lower than a maximal biological meaningful limit $-C'_i$ (for under-expression). Liu and Chow (2008) proposed that the hypothesis for identifying differentially expressed genes between the tested and controlled conditions can be formulated as the following hypotheses:

$$H_0: -C'_i \leq \mu_{Ti} - \mu_{Ci} \leq C_i$$

versus

$$H_1: \mu_{Ti} - \mu_{Ci} < -C'_i \quad \text{or} \quad \mu_{Ti} - \mu_{Ci} > C_i, \quad i = 1, \ldots, G$$

It should be noted that the biologically meaningful fold changes are different among the genes. In addition, many important, biologically significant, differentially expressed genes may have very subtle fold changes, which may be smaller than a twofold change (Hughes et al., 2000). Liu and Chow (2008) proposed a two one-sided test procedure based on t-statistics. However, simulation results showed that this procedure may be very conservative. In addition, expression levels of genes are correlated. Consequently, to overcome the conservatism and to take into account the correlation structure of expression levels, Liu et al. (2008) suggested a permutation procedure for the two one-sided hypotheses. Its performance in terms of size and power seems adequate.

The issue of false identification of differentially expressed genes could become very serious and may have a devastating consequence on the diagnostic accuracy and reproducibility of the results. Ma et al. (2004) suggested the use of the ratio of the expression levels of two genes for the prognosis of clinical outcome of the patients with early-stage breast cancer after receiving tamoxifen. However, their findings could not be reproduced by other investigators (Reid et al., 2005). One of the many possible reasons for this is the issue of false-positive rate. These researchers restricted their search to 5457 genes that exhibited a great variation among the 60 laser-capture microdissected samples. At a rather stringent significance level of 0.001, they found statistical significance only in 9 genes. However, as pointed out by Simon (2005), at a significance level of 0.001 for 5457 genes, one would expect to find at least 5.4 (0.001 × 5457) falsely identified genes by chance alone, even though they are in fact not differentially expressed between the test and the control samples. Consequently, the false discovery rate was 0.6 (5.4/9). In other words, 60% of the identified genes could not discriminate the test samples from the control, and its predictability could not be confirmed by independent data.

The number of genes in the original set was statistically and significantly associated with the clinical outcome identified during the development of MammaPrint using 25 k microarrays was 231. Therefore, if the same nominal significance level of 0.001 is applied, 25 statistically significant genes will be identified by chance alone. Therefore, for the initial set, the false discovery rate of 10.8% seems reasonable. However, the MammaPrint includes a reduced set of only 70 genes. This increases the false discovery rate to 35.7%, which may still cause some concerns, despite the fact that the most significant 70 genes were selected in a sequential step of five genes each, and consistent results on analytical performance and clinical utility between the original and reduced sets of genes were demonstrated (Buyse et al., 2006; Glas et al., 2006).

For any device with multiple heritable markers that can be clinically meaningful and whose validation can be practically feasible, it must be represented in a parsimonious manner with a clinically meaningful threshold that can provide the best classification and/or diagnostic accuracy. In fact, these devices with multiple heritable markers are parallel assays with many analytes, and hence, the measurements of these analytes are the expression levels in the same unit. As a result, there are various forms for an overall representation of expression patterns. For example, MammaPrint Index is in fact the correlation coefficient of the sample expression profile with the mean expression profile of 44 tumors with a known good clinical outcome. On the other hand, Ma et al. (2004) employed the ratio of the expression levels of HOXB13 to IL17BR to distinguish relapse patients from the disease-free patients after receiving tamoxifen. The idea of using the correlation coefficient as a prognostic index for MammaPrint is because these 70 genes discriminate the patients without distant metastasis from those with metastasis; therefore, a low estimated correlation coefficient between the expression profile of a test sample with the template of 40 tumors with good clinical outcome predicts a high risk of distant metastasis for the patient. On the other hand, HOXB13 is over-expressed in tamoxifen-treated patients with recurrence, and IL17BR is over-expressed in tamoxifen-treated patients without recurrence. Consequently, a large HOXB13 to IL17BR ratio may indicate a high risk of recurrence for tamoxifen-treated patients, and vice versa.

Although both the correlation coefficient and ratio of expression levels have been applied in some limited clinical studies as useful prognostic devices for clinical outcomes, statistically, their classification properties have not been theoretically investigated. Possible reasons may be that most statistical theories for classification are based on either a single marker or a linear form of multiple markers. With respect to the linear representation of expression levels of multiple heritable markers, Su and Liu (1993) revealed that the Fisher linear discrimination function provides not only the coefficients of the best linear combination, but also the largest area under the generalized ROC curve. However, estimation and testing procedures for comparison of the paired areas under the generalized ROC curves between the two devices have not been fully developed and require further research (Liu and Chow, 2008; Reiser and Faraggi, 1997).

During the early-development stage, differentially expressed genes are identified using all possible genes. However, for a device product developed for routine clinical practice, only a small number of genes will be considered for the inclusion in the device. For example, MammaPrint consists of 1900 60-mer oligonucleotide probes, which account for only 7.6% of the original 25 k. These 1900 features include the 70 genes that have the discrimination power to distinguish patients with high risk of recurrence from those with low risk. On the other hand, despite the different technology platforms, Oncotype DX breast-cancer assay only selects 21 genes. As a result, how many and which genes should be included in the devices still remains a great challenge to the researchers. However, the most important issues are their biological meaning and mechanism for the disease etiology, and their clinical interpretation. If there is unequivocal evidence that a certain biological pathway is involved in the pathogenesis of a disease, all genes affecting this pathway should be included in the device irrespective of whether they are differentially expressed or not. On the other hand, as mentioned before, only a small portion of genes will be identified as differentially expressed. Therefore, during the early stage of development, the exact number of genes that will be included in the final device is not known, and hence, the number of genes included in the final device product is a random variable. It follows that the variability of the number of genes should be considered in validation of the device during the development stage. Statistically, Liu and Chow (2008) suggested that the number of genes and the genes to be included in the device should reach a balance between the practicality and the amount of information required for an accurate diagnosis for the intended use. They also suggested the partial between-group distance (PBGD) as a guide for determination of the number of genes to be included in the device.

8.3.2   Validation Procedures

As for the traditional assay, principles for performance evaluation of diagnostic devices using heritable markers for molecular targets involve analytical and clinical studies. Analytical studies are for quality control and assay validation, while clinical studies are for the utilities, effectiveness, and safety of the devices. Therefore, the primary objectives of validation of any analytical procedures are assessment of accuracy and precision of the devices, which include specificity, linearity, range, repeatability, intermediate precision, reproducibility, detection limit, quantitative limit, and robustness. As described earlier, Oncotype DX used in the TAILORx trial is an RT-PCR assay based on 21 genes, while a 70-gene molecular signature derived from the microarray is used in the MINDACT trial. Therefore, IVDMIAs are parallel assays with multiple biomarkers and multiple medical decision points. Validation of IVDMIA should address the performance and assay validation for each component as well as the overall quality performance of the whole IVDMIAs (Frueh, 2006; Patterson et al., 2006). The FDA guidances on pharmacogenetic tests and gene-expression profiling test systems suggest that for each target or expression pattern, the performance characteristics include assay sensitivity, reproducibility, validation of cutoff, reference range or medical decision point, assay range, and specificity (FDA, 2007a,b). The FDA guidances also recommend consulting with the guidelines on protocols for assay validation in clinical laboratory published by the Clinical Laboratory Standard Institutes (CLSI). However, these protocols are for a single analyte and are not suitable for complicated assay with multiple markers and multiple statistical algorithms for prognosis or diagnosis. As a result, the assay validation of IVDMIAs should employ different approaches, although the principle of accuracy and precision remains the same (Canales et al., 2006; Ji and Davis, 2006).

The overall analytical performance of the device based on multiple heritable markers is determined by the performance of the individual component markers. Therefore, at the minimum, the performance of each single gene should be evaluation by the approved guidelines on validation protocols issued by the CLSI. In addition, the results of individual markers are integrated into a single score or index by some special algorithms whose derivations are not transparent and cannot be independently derived or verified by the end users. For example, based on the expression profile of 21 genes, the Oncotype DX breast-cancer assay provides a recurrence score from 0 to 100 and the MammaPrint yields the MammaPrint Index with a range from -1 to $+1$ before they are converted into a yes/no classification rule. Although the algorithms to derive these scores or indices are not totally transparent, both Oncotype DX recurrence score and MammaPrint Index are quantitative values, and hence, analytical accuracy and precision of the devices can be assessed by and should be focused on these numeric numbers. Therefore, traditional designs for evaluation of repeatability (intra-run precision), inter-run precision, and between-site reproducibility recommended by CLSI Guideline EP5-A2 should be employed for these scores or indices (CLSI, 2004). On the other hand, these devices are based on the heritable markers. As a result, the designs for evaluation of accuracy and precision should also consider important factors, such as specimen collection, storage, shipping method, transit time, RNA amount, quality and integrity, dye effect, operators, different batches, and cross-hybridization. The results on analytical accuracy and precision obtained from these studies should be provided in the package inserts.

The summary decision of the MammaPrint indicates that linearity is not applicable for this type of assay, which is not entirely true. Both Oncotype DX breast-cancer assay and MammaPrint transform the gene-expression profile of the sample into a single continuous index, which is supposed to be proportional to the risk of recurrence or distant metastasis for the patient. Therefore, linearity and the assay range are important characteristics of the devices. If the linearity cannot be established, especially at the thresholds, then the prognostic power or predictability of the devices may be seriously in doubt. The main reason is that the reference standards with known risk are not available for the evaluation of linearity in assay validation of IVDMIAs. However, if the reference standards are obtainable and the linearity of IVDMIAs can be assessed and ascertained, not only accuracy of the device is increased, but also the misclassification rate may be reduced.

Since the IVDMIAs are developed and approved for routine clinical practice for either prognosis of risk or prediction of the response to treatment, both the U.S. FDA guidances on pharmacogenetic tests and gene-expression profiling test systems require the sponsors to provide data from clinical studies to support the indication for use and claims of the devices. The following are a summary of general considerations for planning and evaluating clinical studies recommended by the U.S. FDA guidances on pharmacogenetics tests and gene-expression profiling test systems:

1. Plan studies to support the intended use claim for the device with data that are representative of the population for the intended device.

2. Describe all protocols for internal and external evaluation studies.

3. Clearly define the inclusion and exclusion criteria for the targeted population to which the device is intended.

4. Describe the sampling method used in the selection and exclusion of patients. Ideally, the samples should be collected from the patients enrolled in a prospective, randomized, controlled trial.

5. When archived specimens are used or when a retrospection study is employed, prespecified inclusion/exclusion criteria for samples and justification of relevance of the sampled population to the targeted population for the intended use should be provided.

6. Irrespective of being prospective or retrospective studies, since both these studies are for validation, independent samples must be used. In other words, the sample used for clinical validation must be different and independent of the samples used for development.

7. Establish uniform protocols for all external evaluation sites prior to study initiation and execute the studies consistently according to the protocols throughout the entire duration of the study and data collection.

8. For the clinical validation study, the validation data set should include clinical samples collected from three different clinical sites in different geographical locations. It is preferable that clinical validation studies be conducted within the US population.

9. If clinically or statistically justified, analyze the data for each individual site and pooled over sites. Justification of data pooling over sites should address variation between sites in prevalence, age, gender, and race/ethnicity.

10. Clearly specify the plans to define population-sampling bias.

11. Define clinical truth, which is the best clinical evidence for a specific diagnosis or allele assignment. In addition, the definition of the measure for clinical truth should be provided along with the method by which the measure is obtained.

12. Describe how the cutoff point will initially be set, and how it will be verified. If a cutoff is specified for each of multiple alleles, genotypes, or mutations, the performance characteristics of each cutoff with respect to allele, genotype, or mutation should be described. Statistical methods, such as ROC curve, should be used for the determination of cutoff.

13. Describe the appropriate prognostic/predictive endpoints. Examples are time from surgery to distant metastasis, OS, and DFS.

14. Describe the statistical methods for validation strategy either in the protocol or in the statistical analysis plan. The clinical validation of the MammaPrint used

the hazard ratio to quantify the relative risk of distant metastasis in the high-risk group in comparison with the low-risk group. The expected relative risk as measured in terms of hazard ratio should be representative of a clinically relevant difference that validates a gene signature as a prognostic/predictive index.

15. Determine the sample size prior to beginning the clinical study, preferably in the study protocol. It is highly recommended that the sample size have sufficient power to detect the differences of clinical importance for each marker, mutation, or profile.

16. Account for all individuals and samples.

17. Perform studies using appropriate methods for quality control.

For the prognostic devices, the guidance on gene-expression profiling test system requires prognostic performance to be measured by positive predictive value (PPV) and negative predictive value (NPV). For the prognosis of distant metastasis for early breast cancer after receiving surgery, the PPV is the probability of metastasis within certain years, given that the results yielded by the device are of high risk; while the NPV is the probability of no metastasis within certain years, given that the results yielded by the device are of low risk. The U.S. FDA guidance indicates that 5 years is the minimum time point for the evaluation of distant metastasis for breast cancer. In addition, the evidence of added value of prognosis after considering the current available and standard prognostic clinical factors should be provided. For example, in the clinical validation study, the gene signature provided by the MammaPrint, based on hazard ratio, is proven to be a statistically significant, independent prognostic factor of the risk of distant metastasis, in addition to the clinicopathological criteria (Buyse et al., 2006).

8.4 Discussion and Final Remarks

Although the U.S. FDA guidances on pharmacogenetics tests and gene-expression profiling test systems state the regulatory requirements on the analytical performance and clinical validation, little attention has been paid to the statistical design for clinical investigations. On the other hand, the U.S. FDA draft paper on Drug-Diagnostic Co-Development discusses various designs for clinical utility studies (FDA, 2005). In general, there are two types of the statistical designs. According to Sargent et al. (2005), treatment-by-device interaction design is for predictive markers, which predict the response to therapy. In this design, the patients are stratified by the positive and negative results of the device. Within each stratum, the patients are randomized to receive the test and reference treatments. The same test and reference treatments are used in both strata, because the objective of the design is to identify treatment-by-device interaction. However, if it is known a priori that the test treatment may be efficacious only in positive (or negative) patients, the enrichment design may be employed, for example, the ALTTO trial for directly comparing Herceptin with lapatinib in patients with over-expressed/over-amplified HER gene (The ALTTO trial, 2008). On the other hand, a prognostic device is only to assess a patient's risk of a certain clinical outcome, such as distant metastasis or recurrence of the disease. Therefore, it is for the selection of treatment regimens for the patients. Sargent et al. (2005) suggested a modified device-based strategy design for validation of the prognostic device. In a device-based strategy design, patients are randomized either to use the device or to not to use it. The patients randomized not to use the device will further be randomized to receive either the reference treatment or the test treatment. The patients who are randomized to use the device and have a positive (or negative) result will receive the test (or reference) treatment. This modified device-based design allows us to investigate whether the efficacy of the device-based strategy is due to the true clinical utility of the device or an improvement of therapeutic regimen independent of the test results of the device. Both TAILORx trial and the MINDACT trial adopted this design.

As stated in the U.S. FDA guidance, currently, a gene-expression profiling test system is only of prognostic purpose and it is not intended for diagnosis, or to predict or detect response to therapy, or to help select the optimal therapy for patients. However, the ultimate goal of TM is the individualized treatment for each patient based on the patient's clinical or pharmacogenetics characteristics. For example, the primary objective of the MINDACT trial is to determine whether the patients should receive the unnecessary adjuvant chemotherapy or less aggressive endocrine therapy based on the results of risk obtained from the 70-gene signature provided by the MammaPrint. Therefore, although the MammaPrint currently is approved as a Class II device for prognosis of the risk of distant metastasis, its ultimate utility lies on the selection of the optimal treatment regimen for the early-stage patients. Therefore, it may become a Class III device for prediction of response to therapy.

The U.S. FDA guidance on pharmacogenetic tests and gene-expression profiling test system for breast cancer allows retrospective clinical validation of a device if a full description of selection (inclusion/exclusion) criteria and characterization of relevant features and limitations of the samples are provided. However, in practice, it is rather difficult to achieve these goals. For example, the validation series of the MammaPrint include 403 samples from the patients who were diagnosed over a span of 18 years (1980–1999) with a median follow-up of 13.6 years (Buyse et al., 2006). The diagnostic criteria, timing, and methods for collecting and storing the samples may change rapidly and drastically over 18 years. For example, useful RNA could be extracted for hybridization and analysis only from 326 samples. Thus, variation associated with the technology and medical concept about the diagnosis and treatment of breast cancer over two decades may not be quantified. In addition, missing tumor size and ER status occurred in some patients. As a result, only 302 patients had complete data for validation. It is not clear whether the characteristics of the patients are different between the patients with complete data and those with missing data. Consequently, the extent of the validation bias of the MammaPrint cannot be measured.

As mentioned earlier, the U.S. FDA guidance on gene-expression profiling test system requires evaluation of PPV and NPV. The decision summary for the

MammaPrint reports that it has a PPV value of 0.22 for metastatic disease after 5 years. In other words, 78% of the patients with a positive result by MammaPrint will not have metastatic disease after 5 years. This implies that 78% of the patients will receive unnecessary adjuvant chemotherapy with possible serious adverse effects. One of the possible explanations is that multivariate methods, such as the Cox proportional hazard model, were not employed to investigate the additional contributions by the 70-gene signature, owing to the reason for avoiding the possible multicollinearity among variables. In addition, the improvement on prognostic accuracy of the MammaPrint over clinicopathological criteria as measured by the area under the ROC curve was found to be only 2.2%, which is quite small. This phenomenon shows that it cannot be used alone and should probably be applied in conjunction with currently available validated prognostic factors. As a result, in the decision summary and package insert, the results of added prognostic/diagnostic accuracy should be reported, preferably using the area of the ROC curves, In addition, the performance on clinical accuracy should be reported for the device alone and for the device in combination with other validated prognostic factors.

References

The ALTTO trial. 2008. http://www.cancer.gov/. Accessed on March 1, 2008.

Buyse, M., Loi, S., van't Veer, L., et al. 2006. Validation and clinical utility of a 70-gene prognostic signature for women with node-negative breast cancer. *Journal of the National Cancer Institute*, 98, 1183–1192.

Benjamini, Y. and Hochberg, Y. 1995. Controlling the false discovery rate: A practical and powerful approach to multiple testing. *Journal of Royal Statistical Society, Series B* 57, 289–300.

Canales, R.D., Luo, Y., Willey, J.C., et al. 2006. Evaluation of DNA microarray results with quantitative gene expression platforms. *Nature Biotechnology*, 24, 1115–1122.

Casciano, D.A. and Woodcock, J. 2006. Empowering microarrays in the regulatory setting. *Nature Biotechnology*, 24, 1103.

Chow, S.C. and Liu, J.P. *Statistical Design and Analysis in Pharmaceutical Statistics*. Marcel Dekker Inc., New York, 1995.

CLSI. Approved Guideline EP5-A2, *Evaluation of Precision Performance of Quantitative Measurement Methods*, Clinical Laboratory Standard Institute, Wayne, PA, 2004.

Dalton, W.S. and Friend, S.H. 2006. Cancer biomarkers—An invitation to the table. *Science*, 312, 1165–1168.

Dudoit, S., Yang, Y.H., Callow, M.J., and Speed, T.P. 2002. Statistical methods for identifying differentially expressed genes in replicated cDNA microarray experiments. *Statistica Sinica*, 12, 111–139.

FDA. Decision Summary P040030, Rockville, Maryland, USA, 2004.

FDA. Draft concept paper on *Drug-Diagnostic Co-Development*, Rockville, Maryland, 2005.

FDA. Guidance on *Gene Expression Profiling Test System for Breast Cancer Prognosis*, Rockville, Maryland, 2007a.

FDA. Guidance on *Pharmacogenetic Tests and Genetic Tests for Heritable Markers*, Rockville, Maryland, 2007b.

FDA. Draft Guidance on *In Vitro Diagnostic Multivariate Index Assays*, Rockville, Maryland, 2007c.

FDA. Guidance on *Statistical Guidance on Reporting Results from Studies Evaluating Diagnosis Tests*, Rockville, Maryland, 2007d.

FDA. Decision Summary k062694, Rockville, Maryland, 2007e.

Frueh, F.W. 2006. Impact of microarray data quality on genomic data submissions to the FDA. *Nature Biotechnology*, 24, 1105–1107.

Glas, A.M., Floor, A., Delahaye, LJMJ, et al. 2006. Converting a breast microarray signature into a high-throughput diagnostic test. *BMC Genomics* 7, 278.

Hochberg, Y. and Tamhane, A.C. *Multiple Comparison Procedures*, Wiley, New York, 1987.

Hughes, T.R., Marton, M.J., Jones, A.R., et al. 2000. Functional discovery via a compendium of expression profiles. *Cell*, 102, 109–126.

Ji, H. and Davis, R.W. 2006. Data quality in genomics and microarray. *Nature Biotechnology*, 24, 1112–1113.

Li, C.R., Liao, C.T., and Liu, J.P. 2008. A non-inferiority test for diagnostic accuracy based on the paired partial areas under ROC curves, *Statistics in Medicine*, 27, 1762–1776.

Liu, J.P. and Chow, S.C. 2008. Statistical issues on the diagnostic multivariate index assay and targeted clinical trials, *Journal of Biopharmaceutical Statistics*, 18, 167–182.

Liu, J.P., Liao, C.T., Chiu, S.T., and Dai, J.Y. 2008. A permutation two one-sided tests procedure to test minimal fold changes of gene expression levels. *Journal of Biopharmaceutical Statistics*, in press.

Ma, X., Wang, Z., Ryan, P.D., et al. 2004. A two-gene expression ratio predicts clinical outcome in breast cancer patients treated with tamoxifen. *Cancer Cell*, 5, 607–616.

MINDACT Design and MINDACT trial overview. http://www.breastinternational group.org/transbig.html. Accessed on June 5, 2006.

Paik, S., Shak, S., Tang, G., et al. 2004. A multigene assay to predict recurrence of tamoxifen-treated, node-negative breast cancer. *New England Journal of Medicine*, 351, 2817–2826.

Paik, S., Tang, G., Shak, S., et al. 2006. Gene expression and benefit of chemotherapy in women with node-negative, estrogen receptor-positive breast cancer. *Journal of Clinical Oncology*, 24, 1–12.

Patterson, T.A., Lobenhofer, E.K., Fulmer-Smentek, S.B., et al. 2006. Performance comparison of one-color and two-color platforms with the MAQC project. *Nature Biotechnology*, 24, 1140–1150.

Ravdin, P.M., Siminoff, L.A., Davis, G.J., et al. 2001. Computer program to assist in making of decision about adjuvant therapy for women with early breast cancer. *Journal of Clinical Oncology*, 19, 980–991.

Reid, J.F., Lusa, L., De Cecco, L., et al. 2005. Limits of predictive models using microarray data for breast cancer treatment clinical outcome. *Journal of National Cancer Institute*, 97, 927–930.

Reiser, B. and Faraggi, D. 1997. Confidence intervals for the general ROC criterion. *Biometrics*, 53, 644–652.

Sargent, D.J., Conley, B.A., Allegra, C., and Collette, L. 2005. Clinical trial designs for predictive marker validation in cancer treatment trials, *Journal of Clinical Oncology*, 23, 2020–2027.

Simon, R.M. 2005. Development and validation of therapeutic relevant multi-gene biomarker classifier, *Journal of the National Cancer Institute*, 97, 866–867.

Simon, R.M., Korn, E.L., McShane, L.M., Radmacher, M.D., Wright, G.W., and Zhao, Y. *Design and Analysis of DNA Microarray Investigations*. Springer, New York, 2003.

Sprarano, J., Hayes, D, Dees, E., et al. 2006. Phase III randomized study of adjuvant combination chemotherapy and hormonal therapy versus adjuvant hormonal therapy alone in women with previously resected axillary node-negative breast cancer with various levels of risk for recurrence (TAILORx trial). http://www.cancer.gov/clinicaltrials/ECOG-PACCT-1. Accessed on June 5, 2006.

Su, J.Q. and Liu, J.S. 1993. Linear combination of multiple diagnostic markers. *Journal of the American Statistical Association*, 88, 1350–1355.

Swain, S.M. 2006. A step in the right direction. *Journal of Clinical Oncology*, 24(23), 1–2.

Tusher, V.G., Tibshirani, R., and Chu, G. 2001. Significance analysis of microarrays applied to ionizing radiation response. *Proceedings of National Academy of Sciences*, 98, 5116–5121.

van't Veer, L.J., Dai, H., Van de Vijver, M.J., et al. 2002. Gene expression profiling predicts clinical outcome of breast cancer. *Nature*, 415, 530–536.

Van de Vijver, M.J., He, Y.D., van't Veer, L.J., et al. 2002. A gene-expression signature as a predictor of survival in breast cancer. *New England Journal of Medicine*, 347, 1999–2009.

Varmus, H. 2006. The new era in cancer research. *Science*, 312, 1162–1165.

Wang, S. and Ethier, S. 2004. A generalized likelihood ratio test to identify differentially expressed genes from microarray data. *Bioinformatics*, 20, 100–104.

Chapter 9

Translation in Clinical Information between Populations—Bridging Studies

Chin-Fu Hsiao, Mey Wang, Herng-Der Chern, and Jen-pei Liu

Contents

9.1 Introduction

In recent years, geotherapeutics has attracted much attention from the sponsors as well as regulatory authorities. However, the questions lie on when and how to address the geographic variations of efficacy and safety for the product development. It will strongly depend on the size of the market, development cost, and the factors influencing the clinical outcomes for the evaluation of efficacy and safety. If the size of the market for some new geographic region is sufficiently large, then it is understandable that the sponsor may be willing to repeat the whole clinical development program after the test product has completed its development plan, and maybe obtain the market approval in the original region. Ideally, one of course can directly conduct studies in the new region with sample size similar to the phase III trials conducted in the original region for confirming the efficacy observed in the original region. Nonetheless, extensive duplication of the clinical evaluation in the new region not only demands valuable development resources, but also delays the availability of the test product to the needed patients in the new regions. To address this issue, a general framework is provided by the ICH E5 (1998) document entitled *Ethnic Factors in the Acceptability of Foreign Clinical Data* for evaluation of the impact of the ethnic factors on the efficacy, safety, dosage, and dose regimen.

The ICH E5 guideline suggests that a bridging study (BS) be conducted in the new region to generate additional information to bridge the foreign clinical data, when this data contained in the complete clinical data package (CCDP) cannot provide sufficient bridging evidence. According to the ICH E5 guideline, a BS is therefore defined as a supplementary study conducted in the new region to provide pharmacodynamic or clinical data on the efficacy, safety, dosage, and dose regimen to allow extrapolation of the foreign clinical data to the population of the new region. Recently, interest has developed in assessing the similarity based on the additional information from the BS and the foreign clinical data in the CCDP.

According to the ICH E5 guideline, the ethnic factors are classified into the following two categories: intrinsic and extrinsic factors. Intrinsic ethnic factors are factors that define and identify the population in the new region and maybe influence the ability to extrapolate clinical data between regions. They are more genetic and physiologic in nature, e.g., genetic polymorphism, age, gender, etc. On the other hand, extrinsic ethnic factors are factors associated with the environment and culture. Extrinsic ethnic factors are more social and cultural in nature, e.g., medical practice, diet, and practices in clinical trials and conduct. In addition, the ICH E5 guideline provides regulatory strategies of minimizing duplication of the clinical data and requirement of bridging the evidence for extrapolation of foreign clinical data to a new region.

Several statistical procedures have been proposed to assess the similarity based on the additional information from the BS and the foreign clinical data in the CCDP. Shih (2001) used the method of Bayesian most-plausible prediction for drug approval for countries in the Asia-Pacific region. As substantial information from multicenter studies has already shown efficacy in the original regions (say for example, the United States or the European Union) when a drug manufacturer seeks marketing approval in another new region (say for example, an Asian country), the result from the new region is consistent with the previous results if it falls within the previous experience. Chow et al. (2002) proposed to use reproducibility probability and generalizability to assess the necessity of BS in the new region. Liu et al. (2002) used a hierarchical model approach to incorporate the foreign bridging information into the data generated by the BS in the new region. Lan et al. (2005) introduced the weighted Z-tests in which the weights may depend on the prior observed data for the design of bridging studies.

In this chapter, we will focus on BS for translating clinical information (results) from one region (a population) to another (a different population). In Section 9.2, we will introduce statistical methods to synthesize the data generated by the BS and the foreign clinical data generated in the original region, for assessment of similarity based on superior efficacy of the test product over a placebo control. In Section 9.3, we will introduce the experience of Taiwan on implementing the bridging evaluations. Lastly, some concluding remarks are given in Section 9.4.

9.2   Translation in Different Populations

Nowadays, the increasing evidence that genetic determinants may mediate variability among persons in response to a drug implies that the patients' responses to therapeutics may vary among racial and ethnic groups. In other words, after the intake of identical doses of a given agent, some ethnic groups may have clinically significant side effects, whereas others may show no therapeutic response. An example of such a situation can be seen in the study by Caraco (2004). Caraco pointed out that some of this diversity in rates of response can be ascribed to differences in the rate of drug metabolism, particularly by the cytochrome P-450 superfamily of enzymes. While 10 isoforms of cytochrome P-450 are responsible for the oxidative metabolism of most drugs, the effect of genetic polymorphisms on catalytic activity is most prominent for 3 isoforms—CYP2C9, CYP2C19, and CYP2D6. Among these three, CYP2D6 has been most extensively studied and is involved in the metabolism of about 100 drugs, including β-blockers, antiarrhythmic, antidepressant, neuroleptic, and opioid agents. Several studies revealed that some patients are classified as having "poor metabolism" of certain drugs owing to the lack of CYP2D6 activity. On the other hand, patients having some enzyme activity are classified into three subgroups: those with "normal" activity (or extensive metabolism), those with reduced activity (intermediate metabolism), and those with markedly enhanced activity (ultrarapid metabolism). Most importantly, the distribution of CYP2D6 phenotypes varies with race. For instance, the frequency of the phenotype associated with poor metabolism is 5%–10% in the Caucasian population, but only 1% in the Chinese and Japanese populations.

Another example regarding the impact of ethnic factors on the responses to therapeutics is the epidermal growth-factor receptor (EGFR) tyrosine kinase inhibitor, gefitinib (Iressa). Recently, Iressa was approved in Japan and the United States for the treatment of non-small cell lung cancer (NSCLC). The EGFR is a promising target anticancer therapy, because it is more abundantly expressed in the lung-carcinoma tissue than in the adjacent normal lung. However, clinical trials have revealed significant variability in the response to gefitinib, with higher responses observed in Japanese patients than in a predominantly European-derived population (27.5% vs. 10.4%, in a multi-institutional phase II trial) (Fukuoka et al., 2003). Paez et al. (2004) also demonstrated that somatic mutations of the EGFR were found in 15 of 58 unselected tumors from Japan and 1 of 61 from the United States. Treatment with Iressa causes tumor regression in some patients with NSCLC, more frequently in Japan. Finally, the striking differences in the frequency of EGFR mutation and response to Iressa between Japanese and United States patients raised certain general questions regarding the variations in the molecular pathogenesis of cancer in different ethnic, cultural, and geographic groups.

The ICH E5 guideline provides a general framework for evaluation of the impact of ethnic factors on the efficacy, safety, dosage, and dose regimen and also describes regulatory strategies of minimizing duplication of clinical data, and emphasizes on the requirement of bridging evidence for extrapolation of foreign clinical data to a new region. As we know, a BS is conducted in the new region usually only after the test product is approved for commercial marketing, because of its proven efficacy and safety. Furthermore, it must be noted that the sufficient information on efficacy, safety, dosage, and dose regimen has already been generated in the original region, which is available in the CCDP. This is the crucial reason for the ICH E5 guideline to emphasize on minimizing unnecessary duplication of generating clinical data in the new region. Therefore, one should borrow "strength" from the information on dose response, efficacy, and safety from the CCDP in the original region and incorporate them into the analysis of the additional data obtained from the BS. In this section, empirical Bayesian approaches will be introduced to obtain the data generated by the BS and foreign clinical data generated in the original region, for the assessment of similarity based on superior efficacy of the test product over a placebo control.

9.2.1   Use of Prior Information

For simplicity, we only consider the problem for assessment of similarity on efficacy for comparing a test product and a placebo control. Let X_i and Y_j be certain efficacy responses for patients i and j receiving the test product and the placebo control, respectively, in the new region. For simplicity, both X_is and Y_js are normally distributed with variance σ^2. We assume that σ^2 is known, although it can generally be estimated. Let μ_{NT} and μ_{NP} be the population means of the test and placebo, respectively, and let $\Delta_N = \mu_{NT} - \mu_{NP}$. The subscript N in μ_{NT}, μ_{NP}, and Δ_N indicates the new region. As the test product has already been approved in the original region owing to its proven efficacy against placebo control, if the data collected from the BS in the new region also demonstrate a superior efficacy of the test pharmaceutical over the placebo, then the efficacy observed in the population of the new region is claimed to be similar to that of the original region. This concept of similarity is referred to as the similarity by the positive treatment effect. In other words, this concept of similarity can be evaluated through the following hypothesis:

$$H_0: \Delta_N \leq 0 \quad \text{versus} \quad H_A: \Delta_N > 0. \tag{9.1}$$

Of course, one can directly conduct a BS in the new region with sample size similar to the phase III trials conducted in the original region to provide adequate power to test the above-mentioned hypothesis for the confirmation of the efficacy observed in the original region. However, tremendous resource will be allocated to conduct this type of confirmation bridging the trial in the new region. Even when the sponsor is willing to conduct such a trial, recruitment and length of the trial may be serious problems owing to insufficient number of patients available in some small new regions. In addition, the valuable information about the efficacy, safety, and dosage contained in the CCDP are not fully utilized in the design and analysis of the BS. Furthermore, it is extremely critical to incorporate the information of the foreign clinical data into evaluation of the positive treatment effect for the BS conducted in the new region. Liu et al. (2002) proposed a Bayesian approach to use a normal prior to taking up the strength from CCDP for the evaluation of similarity between the new region and the original region. However, their approach would be overwhelmingly dominated by the results of the original region, if there is a serious imbalance in the information provided between the new and original regions. Therefore, instead of the normal prior distribution used in Liu et al. (2002), Hsiao et al. (2007) considered a mixture model for the prior information of Δ_N. Since the prior information used in Liu et al. (2002) is a special case of that used in Hsiao et al. (2007), hereafter, we will only focus on the use of the mixed prior information.

If no information from the CCDP generated in the original region is borrowed, then the test for hypothesis (Equation 9.1) uses the information generated only by the BS conduced in the new region. This is equivalent to assuming a noninformative prior for Δ_N. On the other hand, most of the primary endpoints in a majority of therapeutic areas, such as hypertension, diabetes, and depression, follow or approximately follow a normal distribution. Therefore, it is quite reasonable to use a normal prior for summarization of the results in the CCDP of the original region. As a result, the proposed mixed prior information for Δ_N is a weighted average of two priors as given below

$$\pi(\Delta_N) = \gamma\pi_1(\Delta_N) + (1 - \gamma)\pi_2(\Delta_N), \tag{9.2}$$

where $\pi_1(\cdot) \equiv c$ is a noninformative prior, $\pi_2(\cdot)$ is a normal prior with mean θ_0 and variance σ_0^2, and $0 \le \gamma \le 1$. Since $\pi_1(\cdot)$ is a noninformative prior, c can be any number. Our experience shows that changes in c will not have any influence on the conclusion. Here, for simplicity, c is set to be 1, and π_2 is a normal prior that summarizes the foreign clinical data about the treatment difference provided in the CCDP. In the study by Hsiao et al. (2007), there are two other choices of π_1. Here, $\gamma = 0$ indicates that the prior π is equivalent to the prior used in Liu et al. (2002), while $\gamma = 1$ indicates that no strength of the evidence for the efficacy of the test product relative to the placebo provided by the foreign clinical data in the CCDP from the original region would be borrowed. The choice of weight, γ, should reflect the relative confidence of the regulatory authority on the evidence provided by the BS conducted in the new region versus those provided by the original region. It should be determined by the regulatory authority of the new region by considering the difference in both intrinsic and extrinsic ethnical factors between the new and original regions.

Let n_T and n_P represent the numbers of patients studied for the test product and the placebo, respectively, in the new region. Based on the clinical responses from the BS in the new region, Δ_N can be estimated by

$$\hat{\Delta}_N = \bar{x}_N - \bar{y}_N,$$

where $\bar{x}_N = \sum_{i=1}^{n_T} x_i / n_T$ and $\bar{y}_N = \sum_{j=1}^{n_P} y_j / n_P$. The marginal density of $\hat{\Delta}_N$ is

$$m(\hat{\Delta}_N) = \gamma + (1 - \gamma) \frac{1}{\sqrt{2\pi(\sigma_0^2 + \tilde{\sigma}^2)}} \exp\left\{ -\frac{(\hat{\Delta}_N - \theta_0)^2}{2(\sigma_0^2 + \tilde{\sigma}^2)} \right\}, \tag{9.3}$$

where $\tilde{\sigma}^2 = \sigma^2/n_T + \sigma^2/n_P$. From the given bridging data and prior distribution, the posterior distribution of Δ_N can be determined as

$$\pi(\Delta_N | \hat{\Delta}_N) = \frac{1}{m(\hat{\Delta})} \left\{ \gamma \frac{1}{\sqrt{2\pi}\tilde{\sigma}} \exp\left[-\frac{(\Delta_N - \hat{\Delta}_N)^2}{2\tilde{\sigma}^2} \right] \right.$$
$$\left. + (1 - \gamma) \frac{1}{\sqrt{2\pi}\sigma_0\tilde{\sigma}} \exp\left[-\frac{(\Delta_N - \theta_0)^2}{2\sigma_0^2} - \frac{(\Delta_N - \hat{\Delta}_N)^2}{2\tilde{\sigma}^2} \right] \right\}.$$

With the data from the BS and prior information, similarity on the efficacy in terms of a positive treatment effect for the new region can be established if the posterior probability of similarity

$$P_{SP} = P(\mu_{NT} - \mu_{NP} > 0 | \text{bridging data and prior})$$

$$= \int_0^\infty \pi(\Delta_N | \hat{\Delta}_N) d\Delta_N > 1 - \alpha,$$

for some prespecified $0 < \alpha < 0.5$. However, α is determined by the regulatory agency of the new region and should generally be <0.2 to ensure that posterior probability of similarity is at least 80%.

Let n_N represent the numbers of patients studied per treatment in the new region. Based on the discussion in the previous section, the marginal density of $\hat{\Delta}_N$ in Equation 9.3 can be reexpressed as

$$m(\hat{\Delta}_N) = \gamma + (1 - \gamma) \frac{1}{\sqrt{2\pi(\sigma_0^2 + 2\sigma^2/n_N)}} \exp\left\{ -\frac{(\hat{\Delta}_N - \theta_0)^2}{2(\sigma_0^2 + 2\sigma^2/n_N)} \right\}.$$

The posterior distribution of Δ_N is, therefore, given by

$$\pi(\Delta_N | \hat{\Delta}_N) = \frac{1}{m(\hat{\Delta})} \left\{ \gamma \frac{1}{\sqrt{4\pi\sigma^2/n_N}} \exp\left[-\frac{(\Delta_N - \hat{\Delta}_N)^2}{4\sigma^2/n_N} \right] \right.$$

$$\left. + (1 - \gamma) \frac{1}{\sqrt{4\pi\sigma_0^2\sigma^2/n_N}} \exp\left[-\frac{(\Delta_N - \theta_0)^2}{2\sigma_0^2} - \frac{(\Delta_N - \hat{\Delta}_N)^2}{4\sigma^2/n_N} \right] \right\}.$$

With the given α, θ_0, σ_0^2, σ^2, and the estimate $\hat{\Delta}_N$, we can determine the sample size n_N by finding the smallest n_N, such that the equation

$$P_{SP} = \int_0^\infty \pi(\Delta_N | \hat{\Delta}_N) d\Delta_N > 1 - \alpha$$

is satisfied. Methods for sample-size determination for the BS can be obtained in the study of Hsiao et al. (2007).

9.2.2 Example

For the purpose of illustration, we now hypothesize an example based on our experience from the literature review. In one such case, the CCDP provides the results of three randomized, placebo-controlled trials for a new antidepressant (test drug) conducted in the original region. The design, inclusion, exclusion criteria, dose, and duration of these three trials are similar, and hence, the three trials constituted the pivotal trials for approval in the original region. The primary endpoint was the change from baseline of sitting diastolic blood pressure (mmHg) at week 12. Since the regulatory agency in the new region still had some concerns in the ethnical differences, both intrinsically and extrinsically, a BS was conducted in the new region to compare the difference in the efficacy between the new and original regions. Three scenarios are considered in this example. The first scenario presents the situation where no statistically significant difference in the primary endpoint exists between the test drug and placebo (2-sided p-value $= 0.6430$). The second situation is that the mean reduction of sitting diastolic blood pressure at week 12 of the test drug is statistically significantly greater than the placebo group (2-sided p-value <0.0001). The third scenario is the situation where owing to the insufficient sample size of the BS, no statistical significance is observed between the test drug and the placebo, although the magnitude of the difference between the test drug and placebo observed in the original region is preserved in the new region (2-sided p-value $= 0.0716$). The number of patients and mean reduction and standard deviations of sitting diastolic blood pressure are provided in Table 9.1. The three scenarios are denoted as New 1 (Example 1), New 2 (Example 2), and New 3 (Example 3), respectively. The alternative hypothesis of interest is that the difference in change from baseline in the sitting diastolic blood pressure at week 12 between the test drug and placebo is <0.

TABLE 9.1:   Descriptive statistics of reduction from baseline in sitting diastolic blood pressure (mmHg).

		Treatment Group	
Region	Statistics	Drug	Placebo
Original 1	N	138	132
	Mean	-18	-3
	Standard deviation	11	12
Original 2	N	185	179
	Mean	-17	-2
	Standard deviation	10	11
Original 3	N	141	143
	Mean	-15	-5
	Standard deviation	13	14
New 1 (Example 1)	N	64	65
	Mean	-4.7	-3.8
	Standard deviation	11	11
New 2 (Example 2)	N	64	65
	Mean	-15	-2
	Standard deviation	11	11
New 3 (Example 3)	N	24	23
	Mean	-11	-4
	Standard deviation	13	13

TABLE 9.2: Values of P_{SP} derived from examples 1, 2, and 3 with various values of γ.

	P_{SP}		
γ	**Example 1**	**Example 2**	**Example 3**
0.0	≈ 1.0000	≈ 1.0000	≈ 1.0000
0.1	0.6789	0.9999	0.9727
0.2	0.6789	0.9999	0.9700
0.3	0.6789	0.9999	0.9690
0.4	0.6789	0.9999	0.9685
0.5	0.6789	0.9999	0.9682
0.6	0.6789	0.9999	0.9680
0.7	0.6789	0.9999	0.9678
0.8	0.6789	0.9999	0.9677
0.9	0.6789	0.9999	0.9676
1.0	0.6789	0.9999	0.9675

Using the technique of meta-analysis (Petitti, 2000) to integrate the results from all the original regions, we derive that $\theta_0 = -13.91$ and $\sigma_0^2 = 0.59$. For the first two scenarios of the BS considered here, $\hat{\sigma}^2 = 3.75$ for the estimation of $\tilde{\sigma}^2$, while $\hat{\sigma}^2 = 14.39$ for the estimation of $\tilde{\sigma}^2$ in the last scenario. Table 9.2 provides the values of P_{SP} with various values of γ for all the three scenarios. For Example 1, the difference in the mean reduction of sitting blood pressure between the test drug and the placebo is 0.9 mmHg, which is strikingly different from those obtained from the three trials conducted in the original region. If the regulatory agency allows all the information of the original region to be used for the evaluation of similarity between the new and original regions, γ is set to be 0 and hence $P_{SP} \approx 1.00$, which are the same results obtained by Liu et al. (2002). Therefore, we conclude that the efficacy observed in the BS of the new region in terms of a positive treatment effect is similar to the efficacy from the original region, even if there is no statistically significant difference in the primary endpoint between the test drug and placebo. This phenomenon implies that when all information from the original region is used, the results of the BS will be overwhelmingly dominated by those of the original region. On the other hand, if $\gamma \geq 0.1$, then P_{SP} always drops to around 0.6789. Accordingly, we cannot conclude that the results of the new region are similar to those of the original region, if $1 - \alpha$ is set to be $>80\%$. In this case, our proposed procedure reaches a conclusion that is more consistent with the evidence provided by the new region.

On the other hand, for Example 2, the difference in the mean reduction of sitting blood pressure between the test drug and the placebo is 13 mmHg, which is quite consistent with those obtained from the three trials conducted in the original region. As expected, the values of P_{SP} in Example 2 appear to be close to 1.00, regardless of the choice of γ. We can thus conclude the similarity between the new and original regions. Again, our procedure reaches a conclusion that is consistent with the evidence provided by the results of the BS conducted in the new region.

For Example 3, the magnitude of the mean difference is 7, which is similar to that of the original region. However, the difference is not statistically significant at the 5% level owing to the smaller sample size and larger variability. As can be observed from Table 9.2, the values of P_{SP} are all >0.9675 for all the values of γ between 0 and 1. Hence, similarity between the new and the original regions is concluded if α is $<10\%$. With the strength of the substantial evidence of efficacy borrowed from the CCDP of the original region, our procedure can prove the similarity of efficacy between the new and the original regions when a nonsignificant efficacy result with a similar magnitude is observed in the BS.

This example demonstrates that with proper selection of γ by the regulatory agency of the new region, the Bayesian approach with the mixture prior in Equation 9.2 reaches a conclusion that is much more in line with the results of the BS in the new region. In addition, the use of mixed prior can avoid the difficulty arising from the imbalance amount of information between the two regions, which is an issue endured by the Bayesian procedure proposed by Liu et al. (2002).

9.3   Implementation of Bridging Study Evaluation in Taiwan

Taiwan government has identified biotechnology as one of the key technologies for Taiwan in the twenty-first century, and biopharmaceutical industry as the most vital and important industry to succeed the semiconductor industry in Taiwan. Owing to the intrinsic and extrinsic factors, the current Taiwan's registration trials cannot adequately address the issue of extrapolation of the results from the original regions to the Taiwan's population. Ideally, the acceptance and exchange of inter-population clinical data between the Caucasian and Asian should be bidirectional. However, in the past, little or no Asian clinical data has been provided in the NDA dossier submitted to the regulatory authorities in Asia. Usually, Caucasian clinical data were the major component of the Clinical Data Package and were automatically accepted as the basis for approval for most of the new drugs in Asia. This situation has been attributed to the small individual markets, weak regulatory authorities, primitive local industries, and poor supporting infrastructure. Recently, after recognizing the ICH E5 concepts and the regional needs for Asian data, countries including Japan, Korea, and Taiwan are showing ever-increasing interest in implementing BS as a part of the requirement for the approval of new drugs.

In general, Taiwan accepts all Asian data. A study by Lin et al. in 2001 determined that the so-called Taiwanese, accounting for 91% of the total population in Taiwan, comprised Minnan and Hakka people who are closely related to the southern Han, and are clustered with other southern Asian populations, such as Thai and Malaysian in terms of HLA typing. Those who are the descendants of northern Han are separated from the southern Asian cluster, and form a cluster with the other northern Asian populations, such as Korean and Japanese. The Taiwanese regulatory authority, therefore, accepts data from trials conducted in Taiwan as well as in other Asian countries, if those trials meet Taiwanese regulatory standards and were conducted in compliance with good clinical practice (GCP) requirements.

From Taiwan's regulatory point of view, ethnic factor should not be defined completely by "Citizenship" or "Race." In the evaluation of ethnic differences, "Drug Characteristics" and "Indication" should be the two major elements to be considered. For example, some medicines are metabolized by the enzymes with genetic polymorphism. If there are higher percentages of poor metabolizers in the Taiwanese patient population for a particular drug, the different assessment models in the risk–benefit ratio and risk management may become necessary. Usually, hepato-toxicity is one of the major safety concerns in the bridging assessment in Taiwan. Owing to the high prevalence rate (18%–20%) of HBsAg carriers in Taiwan, the need for more experiences with the usage of agents with liver toxicity in hepatitis B or C carriers may lead to the necessity of an additional BS. Difference in the disease epidemiology and disease manifestations is another important issue. As in the case with female postmenopausal syndrome, Caucasian women usually present more vasomotor symptoms in contrast to the Taiwanese women, in whom the vasomotor symptoms are not predominant. Therefore, new agents whose efficacy was demonstrated by improved Kupperman Index score (which put more weight on the vasomotor-symptom domain) may not be accepted completely. Further investigations on Taiwanese postmenopausal women, using an index scale more suitable for this population (i.e., Greene Climateric Scale), may be needed. Furthermore, medical practice among the regions usually reflects one of the greatest variation and is the most difficult to harmonize. The GCP compliance, differences in diagnostic criteria for some diseases, potential of drug abuse, and possible drug–drug interactions are all essential considerations in the evaluation for BS.

Taiwan implements the bridging strategy in a stepwise manner. In 1993, the Department of Health (DOH) of Taiwan issued an announcement (the Double-Seven Announcement) for the requirement of including data from local (Taiwan) clinical trials in the NDA dossier for every new medicine seeking marketing approval in Taiwan. The clinical trial should provide data on at least 40 evaluable study subjects, and preferably be randomized, double blinded, and controlled. Subsequently, the DOH issued guidelines on GCP in 1996 and initiated on-site Clinical Trial GCP Inspection in 1999. The standard and quality of local clinical trials improved significantly over time.

Considering the requirement of tremendous financial and human resources in carrying out clinical trials, special or unmet medical needs, practical difficulty with trials in certain diseases, and the desire to minimize duplication of similar or unnecessary trials, the DOH issued five successive announcements of clinical trial waiver between 1998 and 2000. Local clinical trials of drugs in the following nine categories may be waived with no requirement to verify ethnic insensitivity. These include (1) drugs for treatment of AIDS, (2) drugs for organ transplantation, (3) topical agents, (4) nutrition supplements, (5) cathartics used prior to surgery, (6) radio-labeled diagnostic pharmaceuticals, (7) the only choice of treatment for a given serious disease, (8) drugs with demonstrated breakthrough efficacy for life-threatening disease, and (9) drugs for the treatment of rare diseases, where it is difficult to enroll enough subjects for the trial. However, for drugs in a few other categories, the trials may also be waived if the sponsor can provide adequate and proper evidence that the compound is not sensitive to ethnic factors.

On December 12, 2000, the DOH issued an announcement (the Double-Twelve Announcement) for the requirement of including BS report or the protocol in NDA dossier and recommended that the sponsors, before submitting the CCDP to the DOH, apply for a Bridging Study Evaluation (BSE) to assess the necessity for carrying out a BS in Taiwan. The DOH, with help of its Center for Drug Evaluation (CDE), also developed and published a sponsor self-evaluation checklist for BSE to help the sponsors organize pertinent documents for this review. During the transitional period between January 2001 and December 2003, a sponsor could choose to follow the Double-Seven Announcement and perform a clinical trial, or follow the Double-Twelve Announcement and carry out a BSE, then perform a meaningful, well-designed BS, if required. By January 1, 2004, BSE was thoroughly implemented.

From 2001 to 2007, a total of 320 applications of BSE was received and evaluated by the DOH. Among the 280 applications with completed assessment, the percentage of clinical trial waiving was 59.3%. Inadequate or insufficient data on pharmacokinetics (42%), efficacy (31%), and safety (29%) were the most common reasons for which the local clinical trials in Taiwan could not be waived. Eighty-one percent of the cases that failed to obtain a waiver of a BS were new chemical entities, especially drugs with new mechanisms but with little Asian data available. Follow-up analyses indicated that for those cases in which a BS in Taiwan was required, approximately 20% conducted a local trial as requested, and, in approximately 24% of the cases, the sponsor chose to resubmit a more detailed BS package for reevaluation instead of conducting a trial. Among these cases, more than a half failed again to obtain the waiver. For those failure cases, 44% had no follow-up actions.

The following two cases are good examples that well demonstrate the significance of BSE and the plausibility of this bridging strategy in Taiwan. Drug A is a fixed combination of two antiplatelet agents indicated for secondary prevention of thromboembolic stroke. Both the components of the drug had been marketed in Taiwan for a long time. We assessed this new combination with standard BSE procedures and decided to request for a BS, owing to a concern of difference in medical practices (i.e., using a much lower dose for one of the components in Taiwan) and previous AE (headache) experience among Filipinos. The sponsor carried out a BS in Taiwan as requested and the results confirmed our concern. It revealed that the headache-associated dropout rate of patients receiving half dosage for 2 weeks subsequently shifting to full dosage was significantly lower than those receiving full dosage throughout the whole treatment period. The sponsor recognized the ethnic issue from this finding and revised the instruction for use in the LABELING, recommending a lower starting dosage at the first 2 weeks in Asians.

Another drug, B, a powerful new lipid-lowering agent, is metabolized primarily by hepatic CYP2C9 and CYP2C19 (two of the famous polymorphic enzymes in Chinese). According to the Japanese PK study, C_{max} in Japanese was $1.9 \sim 2.5\times$ than in Caucasian, while AUC was $2 \sim 2.5\times$. Although the interracial variability was not huge, we recommended approving the drug with reduced starting and maximal dosage owing to the concern of the rare dose-dependent SAE (i.e., rhabdomyolysis) caused by this drug. This decision was further reflected by the FDA of the United

States. In March 2005, after reviewing the results of a phase IV PK study in Asian-Americans, FDA urged the sponsor to reduce the starting dose of Asians and modify the LABELING accordingly.

The requirement of BS has ushered a new paradigm for regulatory approval in Taiwan. Previous administrative regulation, such as the requirement to carry out small-scale local registration trial for all new drugs and free sale certificates were gradually phased out. With the implementation of ICH E5, accompanied by the establishment of sound IND consultation processes and practice of good regulatory sciences, Taiwan has become a preferred site to participate in the global R&D. Phase I–III multinational clinical trials comprising 75.6% (127/168) of all new-drug clinical trials in 2007. These efforts would ultimately benefit the health of the population in Taiwan.

9.4   Concluding Remarks

Empirical Bayesian methods developed by Liu et al. (2002) seem reasonable to derive the data from both the BS and the original region study, for the assessment of bridging evidence. Since a medicine was approved in the original region owing to its substantial evidence of efficacy and safety based on a sufficiently large sample size, the results of the BS using empirical Bayes approach will be overwhelmingly dominated by the results of the original region, owing to an imbalance of sample sizes between the regions. In other words, it is very difficult, if not impossible, to reverse the results observed in the original region, even if the result of the BS is completely opposite. Therefore, Hsiao et al. (2007) developed a Bayesian approach with the use of mixed prior information for the assessment of similarity between the new and original regions, based on the concept of positive treatment effect. The mixed prior information is a weighted average of a noninformative prior and a normal prior. With an appropriate choice of weight, γ, the evaluation of similarity based on the integrated results of the BS in the new region and those from the original region will no longer be overwhelmingly dominated by the results of the original region, owing to an imbalance of sample sizes between the regions. Therefore, the proposed procedure can avoid the situation of concluding similarity between the new and original regions, when the efficacy result of the test drug observed in the BS of the new region is same as or even worse than that of the placebo group. However, as demonstrated in the example, similarity between the new and original regions will be concluded when the difference in primary endpoint between the test drug and placebo observed in the BS is of the same magnitude as that obtained from the original region, although it may not be statistically significant owing to the small sample size of the BS. As a result, our proposed procedure not only can reach a conclusion that is more consistent with the results obtained from the BS, but can also achieve the objective of minimizing duplication of clinical evaluation in the new region as specified in the ICH E5 guidance.

Selection of weight γ by the regulatory agency in the new region should consider all the differences in both intrinsic and extrinsic ethnical factors between the new and original regions and at the same time, should also reflect their belief on the evidence of efficacy provided in the CCDP of the original region. As mentioned earlier, a BS is conducted in the new region because of the concerns on ethnic differences between the new and original regions; therefore, it is suggested that weight $\gamma > 0$. However, from the example, it can be observed that the weight has a very minimal effect on the sample size of the BS and P_{SP} once it is >0.2. For instance, in Example 1, P_{SP} drops to 0.8 when $\gamma = 1.0E - 0.8$. In other words, even with the use of very little information from the new region, our proposed procedure reaches a conclusion that is more consistent with the evidence provided by the new region.

On the other hand, even if both the regions have positive treatment effect, their effect sizes might in fact be different. That is, their approach could not truly assess the similarity between the two regions. Liu et al. (2004), therefore, proposed a Bayesian approach for assessment of similarity between the new and original regions, based on the concept of noninferiority. Under the noninferiority concept, the efficacy observed in the BS in the new region can be claimed to be similar to that of the original region, if it is no worse than the efficacy of the original region by some clinically acceptable limit. Thus, some difficulties arise using the Bayesian method. First, the Bayesian methods for the evaluation of probability for error of decision making on similarity still require to be worked out. This error probability is extremely crucial for the regulatory authority in the new region to approve a medicine in their jurisdiction. Second, for Bayesian methods, the foreign clinical data provided in the CCDP from the original region and those from the BS in the new region are not generated in the same study and are not internally valid. Hence, a group sequential method (Hsiao et al., 2003) and a two-stage design (Hsiao et al., 2005) were proposed to overcome this issue of internal validity.

References

Caraco, Y. 2004. Genes and the response to drugs. *New England Journal of Medicine*, 351(27), 2867–2869.

Chow, S. C., Shao, J., and Hu, O. Y. P. 2002. Assessing sensitivity and similarity in bridging studies. *Journal of Biopharmaceutical Statistics*, 12, 385–400.

Fukuoka, M., Yano, S., Giaccone, G., Tamura, T., Nakagawa, K., Douillard, J. Y., Nishiwaki, Y., Vansteenkiste, J., Kudoh, S., Rischin, D., Eek, R., Horai, T., Noda, K., Takata, I., Smit, E., Averbuch, S., Macleod, A., Feyereislova, A., Dong, R. P., and Baselga, J. 2003. Multi-institutional randomized phase II trial of gefitinib for previously treated patients with advanced non-small-cell lung cancer. *Journal of Clinical Oncology*, 21(12), 2237–2246.

Hsiao, C. F., Hsu, Y. Y., Tsou, H. H., and Liu, J. P. 2007. Use of prior information for Bayesian evaluation of bridging studies. *Journal of Biopharmaceutical Statistic*, 17(1), 109–121.

Hsiao, C. F., Xu, J. Z., and Liu, J. P. 2003. A group sequential approach to evaluation of bridging studies, *Journal of Biopharmaceutical Statistics*, 13, 793–801.

Hsiao, C. F., Xu, J. Z., and Liu, J. P. 2005. A two-stage design for bridging studies, *Journal of Biopharmaceutical Statistics*, 15, 75–83.

ICH, International Conference on Harmonisation. 1998. *Tripartite Guidance E5 Ethnic Factors in the Acceptability of Foreign Data*. The U.S. Federal Register, 83, pp. 31790–31796.

Lan, K. K., Soo, Y., Siu, C., and Wang, M. 2005. The use of weighted Z-tests in medical research. *Journal of Biopharmaceutical Statistics*, 15(4), 625–639.

Lin, M., Chu, C. C., Chang, S. L., Lee, H. L., Loo, J. H., Akaza, T., Juji, T., Ohashi, J., and Tokunaga, K. 2001. The origin of Minnan and Hakka, the so-called "Taiwanese", inferred by HLA study. *Tissue Antigen*, 57, 192–199.

Liu, J. P., Hsiao, C. F., and Hsueh, H. M. 2002. Bayesian approach to evaluation of bridging studies. *Journal of Biopharmaceutical Statistics*, 12, 401–408.

Liu, J. P., Hsueh, H. M., and Chen, J. J. 2002. Sample size requirement for evaluation of bridging evidence. *Biometrical Journal*, 44, 969–981.

Liu, J. P., Hsueh, H. M., and Hsiao, C. F. 2004. Bayesian non-inferior approach to evaluation of bridging studies. *Journal of Biopharmaceutical Statistics*, 14, 291–300.

Paez, J. G., Janne, P. A., Lee, J. C., Tracy, S., Greulich, H., Gabriel, S., Herman, P., Kaye, F. J., Lindeman, N., Boggon, T. J., Naoki, K., Sasaki, H., Fujii, Y., Eck, M. J., Sellers, W. R., Johnson, B. E., and Meyerson, M. 2004. EGFR mutations in lung cancer: Correlation with clinical response to gefitinib therapy. *Science*, 304(5676), 1497–1500.

Petitti, D. B. 2000. *Meta-Analysis, Decision Analysis, and Cost-Effectiveness Analysis*. Oxford University Press, New York.

Shih, W. J. 2001. Clinical trials for drug registration in Asian-Pacific countries: Proposal for a new paradigm from a statistical perspective. *Controlled Clinical Trials*, 22, 357–366.

Chapter 10

Translation in Clinical Technology— Traditional Chinese Medicine

Chin-Fu Hsiao, Hsiao-Hui Tsou, and Shein-Chung Chow

Contents

10.1 Introduction

Recently, the search for new medicines for treating life-threatening diseases such as cancer has become the center of attention in pharmaceutical research and development. As a result, many pharmaceutical companies have begun to focus on the modernization of traditional Chinese medicines (TCMs). Modernization of TCM is based on scientific evaluations of the efficacy and safety of the TCM, in terms of well-established clinical endpoints for a Western indication through clinical trials on humans. However, it should be recognized that there are fundamental differences in the scientific evaluation of the efficacy and safety of TCM when compared with typical Western medicines (WM), even though they are for the same indication (Chow et al., 2006). In this chapter, we will focus on calibration and validation of the Chinese diagnostic procedure (CDP) with respect to some well-established clinical endpoint (translation in clinical technology). In Section 10.2, we will clarify the difference between TCM and WM; while in Section 10.3, we will introduce the CDP. In Section 10.4, we will discuss the calibration and validation of the CDP for evaluation of TCM with respect to a well-established clinical endpoint for the assessment of WM. Finally, some concluding remarks are given in Section 10.5.

10.2   Differences between TCM and WM

With respect to the medical theory/mechanism, Chinese doctors believe that all the organs within a healthy subject should reach the so-called global dynamic balance or harmony. Once the global balance is broken at certain sites, such as heart, liver, or kidney, some signs and symptoms consequently appear to reflect the imbalance at these sites. An experienced Chinese doctor usually assesses the causes of global imbalance before a TCM with flexible dose is prescribed to fix the problem. With respect to medical practice, we in practice, tend to observe therapeutic effects of WM sooner than TCM. The TCM are often considered for patients who have chronic diseases or non-life-threatening diseases. For critical or life-threatening diseases, TCMs are often used as the second- or third-line treatment with no other alternative treatments. Different medical perceptions regarding the signs and symptoms of certain diseases could lead to a different diagnosis and treatment for the diseases under study. For example, the signs and symptoms of type-2 diabetic subjects could be classified as the disease of thirst reduction by Chinese doctors. However, the disease of type-2 diabetes is not recognized by the Chinese medical literature, although they have the same signs and symptoms as the well-known disease of thirst reduction. This difference in the medical perception and practice has an impact on the diagnosis and treatment of the disease.

TCM treatment typically comprises complicated prescriptions of a combination of several components with certain relative proportions among the components. The component that forms major proportion of the TCM may not be the most active component, while the component that forms the least proportion of the TCM may be the most active component. The relative component-to-component or component-by-food interactions are usually unknown, which may have an impact on the evaluation of clinical efficacy and safety of the TCM. In addition, the use of CDP is to determine what causes the imbalance among these organs. The dose and treatment duration are flexible to achieve the balance point. This concept leads to the so-called personalized medicine, which minimizes the intrasubject variability. On the other hand, most WMs contain a single active ingredient. After drug discovery, an appropriate formulation (or dosage form) is necessarily developed so that the drug can be delivered to the action site in an efficient way. At the same time, an assay is necessarily developed to quantify the potency of the drug product. The drug product is then tested on animals for determining the toxicity and on humans (healthy volunteers) for observing the pharmacological activities.

10.3   Chinese Diagnostic Procedure

TCM is a 3000-year-old medical system encircling the entire scope of human experience. It combines the use of Chinese herbal medicines, acupuncture, massage, and therapeutic exercises (e.g., Qigong [the practice of internal "air"], Taigie, etc.)

for both treatment and prevention of diseases. With its unique theories of etiology, diagnostic systems, and abundant historical literature, TCM itself comprises the Chinese culture and philosophy, clinical practice experiences, and materials including usage experiences of many medical herbs (Wu et al., 2004).

TCM treatment typically comprises complicated prescriptions of a combination of different constituents or components. And the combination is derived based on the CDP. The diagnostic procedure for TCM consists of four major techniques, namely inspection, auscultation and olfaction, interrogation, and pulse taking and palpation. All these diagnostic techniques mainly aim at providing the objective basis for differentiation of syndromes by collecting signs and symptoms from the patients. Inspection involves observing the patient's general appearance (strong or week, fat or thin), mind, complexion (skin color), five sense organs (eye, ear, nose, lip, and tongue), secretions, and excretions. Auscultation involves listening to the voice, expression, respiration, vomit, and cough. Olfaction involves smelling the breath and body odor. Interrogation involves asking questions about specific symptoms and the general condition, including history of the present disease, past history, personal-life history, and family history. Pulse taking and palpation can help to judge the location and nature of a disease according to the changes in the pulse. The smallest detail can have a strong impact on the treatment scheme as well as on the prognosis. While the pulse diagnosis and examination of the tongue receive much attention owing to their frequent mention, the other aspects of the diagnosis cannot be ignored.

After carrying out these four diagnostic techniques, the TCM doctor has to configure a syndrome diagnosis describing the fundamental substances of the body and how they function in the body based on the eight principles, five element theory, five Zang and six Fu, and information regarding the channels and collaterals. The eight principles consist of Yin and Yang (i.e., negative and positive), cold and hot, external and internal, and Shi and Xu (i.e., weak and strong) (Wu, 2000). These eight principles can help the TCM doctors to differentiate the syndrome patterns. For instance, Yin people will develop disease in a negative, passive, and cool way (e.g., diarrhea and back pain), while Yang people will develop disease in an aggressive, active, progressive, and warm way (e.g., dry eyes, tinnitus, and night sweats). The five elements (earth, metal, water, wood, and fire) correspond to particular organs in the human body. Each element operates in harmony with the others.

The five Zang (or Yin organs) includes heart (including the pericardium), lung, spleen, liver, and kidney, while the six Fu (or Yang organs) includes the gall bladder, stomach, large intestine, small intestine, urinary bladder, and the three cavities (i.e., chest, epiastrium, and hypogastrium). Zang organs can manufacture and store fundamental substances. These substances are then transformed and transported by Fu organs. TCM treatments involve a thorough understanding of the clinical manifestations of Zang–Fu organ imbalance and knowledge of appropriate acupuncture points and herbal therapy to rebalance the organs. The channels and collaterals are the representation of the organs of the body. They are responsible for conducting the flow of energy and blood through the entire body.

In addition to providing diagnostic information, these elements of TCM can also help to describe the etiology of the disease, including six exogenous factors (i.e., wind, cold, summer, dampness, dryness, and fire), seven emotional factors (i.e., anger, joy, worry, grief, anxiety, fear, and fright), and other pathogenic factors. Once all this information is collected and processed into a logical and workable diagnosis, the traditional Chinese medical doctor can determine the treatment approach.

10.4   Translation between TCM and WM

For the evaluation of WM, objective criteria based on some well-established clinical study endpoints are usually considered. For example, response rate (CR plus PR based on tumor size) is considered a valid clinical endpoint for evaluating the clinical efficacy of oncology drug products. On the other hand, the CDP for the evaluation of TCM is very subjective. Typically, the CDP consists of four major categories, namely, looking (i.e., inspection), listening and smelling (i.e., auscultation and olfaction), asking (i.e., interrogation), and touching (i.e., pulse taking and palpation). Basically, each category can in fact be thought of as an instrument (or questionnaire) that consists of a number of questions to collect different information regarding patient's activity/function, disease status, or disease severity. An experienced Chinese doctor usually prescribes TCM for the patient based on the combined information obtained from the four major categories along with his/her best judgment. As a result, the relative proportions of the components could vary even with individual patient. In practice, the use of a CDP has raised the following questions: first, it is of interest to determine how accurate and reliable is this subjective diagnostic procedure for evaluation of patients with certain diseases; second, it is also of interest to determine how a change of an observed unit in the CDP be translated to a change in a well-established clinical endpoint for Western indication. We will examine these two questions by studying the calibration and validation of the CDP for evaluation of a TCM with respect to a well-established clinical endpoint for the evaluation of WM.

When planning a clinical trial, it is suggested that the study objectives should be clearly stated in the study protocol. Once the study objectives are confirmed, a valid study design can be chosen and the primary clinical endpoints can be determined accordingly. For evaluation of treatment effect of a TCM, however, the commonly used clinical endpoint is usually not applicable owing to the nature of the CDP, as described earlier. The CDP is in fact an instrument (or questionnaire), which consists of a number of questions to capture the information regarding patient's activity, function, disease status, and severity. As required by most regulatory agencies, such a subjective instrument must be validated before it can be used for assessment of treatment effect in the clinical trials. However, without a reference marker, not only the CDP cannot be validated, but also we do not know whether the TCM has achieved clinically significant effect at the end of the clinical trial. In this section, we will study the calibration and validation of the CDP for evaluation of TCM with respect to a well-established clinical endpoint for the evaluation of WM.

To address these issues, we propose a study design, which allows calibration and validation of a CDP with respect to a well-established clinical endpoint for WM

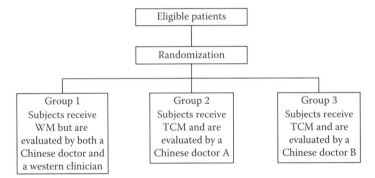

FIGURE 10.1:   Schema of the proposed study design.

(as a reference marker). Subjects will be screened based on criteria for Western indication. Qualified subjects will be diagnosed by the CDP to establish baseline. Qualified subjects will then be randomized to receive either the test TCM or an active control (a well-established Western medicine). The participating physicians, including Chinese doctors and Western clinicians, will also be randomly assigned to either the TCM or the WM arm. Thus, this study design will result in three groups:

Group 1: Subjects who receive WM, but evaluated by both a Chinese doctor and a Western clinician.

Group 2: Subjects who receive TCM and evaluated by a Chinese doctor A.

Group 3: Subjects who receive TCM and evaluated by a Chinese doctor B.

The schema of our proposed study design is shown in Figure 10.1. Group 1 can be used to calibrate the CDP against the well-established clinical endpoint, while Groups 2 and 3 can be used to validate the CDP based on the established standard curve for calibration.

10.4.1   Calibration

Let N be the number of patients in Group 1. For the data from Group 1, let x_j be the measurement of the well-established clinical endpoint of the jth patient. For simplicity, we assume that the measurement of well-established clinical endpoint is continuous. Consider that the TCM diagnostic procedure consists of K items. Let z_{ij} denote the TCM diagnostic score of jth patient from the ith item, $i = 1,\ldots,K$, $j = 1,\ldots,N$. Let y_j represent the scale (or score) of the jth patient summarized from the K TCM diagnostic items. For simplicity, we assume that

$$y_j = \sum_{i=1}^{K} z_{ij}.$$

Similar to calibration of an analytical method (cf. Chow and Liu, 1995), we will consider the five following candidate models:

Model 1: $y_j = \alpha + \beta x_j + e_j$,

Model 2: $y_j = \beta x_j + e_j$,

Model 3: $y_j = \alpha + \beta_1 x_j + \beta_2 x_j^2 + e_j$,

Model 4: $y_j = \alpha x_j^\beta e_j$,

Model 5: $y_j = \alpha e^{\beta x_j} e_j$,

where α, β, β_1, and β_2 are unknown parameters and e's are independent random errors with $E(e_j) = 0$ and finite $\mathrm{Var}(e_j)$ in models 1–3, and $E(\log(e_j)) = 0$ and finite $\mathrm{Var}(\log(e_j))$ in models 4 and 5.

Model 1 is a simple linear regression model, which is probably the most commonly used statistical model for establishment of standard curves for calibration. When the standard curve passes through the origin, model 1 reduces to model 2. Model 3 indicates that the relationship between y and x is quadratic. When there is a nonlinear relationship between y and x, models 4 and 5 are useful. Note that both models 4 and 5 are equivalent to simple linear regression model after logarithm transformation. If all the above models cannot fit the data, generalized linear models can be used.

By fitting an appropriate statistical model between these standards (well-established clinical endpoints) and their corresponding responses (TCM scores), an estimated calibration curve can be obtained. The estimated calibration curve is also known as the standard curve. For a given patient, his/her unknown measurement of well-established clinical endpoint can be determined based on the standard curve, by replacing the dependent variable with its TCM score.

10.4.2   Validity

The validity itself is a measure of bias of the TCM instrument. Since a TCM instrument usually contains the four categories or domains, which in turn consist of a number of questions agreed by the community of the Chinese doctors, it is a great concern that the questions may not be the right questions to capture the information regarding patient's activity/function, disease status, and disease severity. We will use Group 2 to validate the CDP based on the previously established standard curve for calibration. Let X be the unobservable measurement of the well-established clinical endpoint, which can be quantified by the TCM items, Z_i, $i = 1, \ldots, K$ based on the estimated standard curve described in the previous section. For convention, we assume that

$$X = (Y - \alpha)/\beta,$$

where $Y = \sum_{i=1}^{K} Z_i$, i.e., model 1 in Section 10.4.1 was used for calibration. Consider that X is distributed as a normal distribution with mean θ and variance τ^2. Let $Z = (Z_1, \ldots, Z_K)'$. Again, consider that Z follows a distribution with mean

$\mu = (\mu_1,\ldots,\mu_K)'$ and variance Σ. To assess the validity, it is desired to see whether the mean of Z_i, $i = 1,\ldots,K$ is close to $(\alpha + \beta\theta)/K$. Let $\overline{\mu} = \frac{1}{K}\sum_{i=1}^{K}\mu_i$. Then, $\theta = (\overline{\mu} - \alpha)/\beta$. Consequently, we can claim that the instrument is validated in terms of its validity if

$$|\mu_i - \overline{\mu}| < \delta, \quad \forall i = 1,\ldots,K, \tag{10.1}$$

for some small prespecified δ. To verify Equation 10.1, we can consider constructing a simultaneous confidence interval for $\mu_i - \overline{\mu}$. Assume that the TCM instrument is administered to N patients from Group 2. Let $\hat{\mu} = \frac{1}{N}\sum_{j=1}^{N}\mathbf{Z}_j = \bar{\mathbf{Z}}$. Then, the $(1 - \alpha)100\%$ simultaneous confidence interval for $\mu_i - \bar{\mu}$ are given by

$$\mathbf{a}_i'\hat{\mu} - \sqrt{\frac{1}{N}\mathbf{a}_i'S\mathbf{a}_i}T\left(\alpha,K,N-K\right) \leq \mu_i - \bar{\mu} \leq \mathbf{a}_i'\hat{\mu} + \sqrt{\frac{1}{N}\mathbf{a}_i'S\mathbf{a}_i}T\left(\alpha,K,N-K\right),$$

$$i = 1,\ldots\ldots,K,$$

$$\text{where } \mathbf{a}_i' = \begin{pmatrix} -\frac{1}{K}\mathbf{1}_{i-1} \\ 1-\frac{1}{K} \\ -\frac{1}{K}\mathbf{1}_{k-i} \end{pmatrix}, S = \frac{1}{N-1}\sum_{j=1}^{N}\left(\mathbf{Z}_j - \bar{\mathbf{Z}}\right)\left(\mathbf{Z}_j - \bar{\mathbf{Z}}\right)',$$

$$T^2\left(\alpha,K,N-K\right) = \frac{(N-1)K}{N-K}F\left(\alpha,K,N-K\right),$$

and

$$P\left(T^2\left(K,N-K\right) \leq T^2\left(\alpha,K,N-K\right)\right) = 1 - \alpha.$$

The Bonferroni adjustment of an overall α level might be carried out as follows:

$$\mathbf{a}_i'\hat{\mu} - \sqrt{\frac{1}{N}\mathbf{a}_i'S\mathbf{a}_i}T\left(\frac{\alpha}{2K},N-1\right) \leq \mu_i - \bar{\mu} \leq \mathbf{a}_i'\hat{\mu} + \sqrt{\frac{1}{N}\mathbf{a}_i'S\mathbf{a}_i}T\left(\frac{\alpha}{2K},N-1\right).$$

We can reject the null hypothesis that

$$H_0: |\mu_i - \bar{\mu}| \geq \delta, \quad \forall i = 1,\ldots,K, \tag{10.2}$$

if any confidence interval falls completely within $(-\delta,\delta)$.

10.4.3 Reliability

The calibrated well-established clinical endpoints derived from the estimated standard curve are considered reliable, if the variance of X is small. In this regard, we can test the hypothesis

$$H_0: \tau^2 \leq \Delta \text{ for some fixed } \Delta \tag{10.3}$$

to verify the reliability of estimating θ by X. We will use Group 2 to verify the reliability based on the previously established standard curve for calibration. Based on the estimated standard curve, we can derive that

$$\tau^2 = \frac{1}{\beta^2} \text{Var} \left(\sum_{i=1}^{K} Z_i \right)$$

$$= \frac{1}{\beta^2} \mathbf{1}' \Sigma \mathbf{1}.$$

Note that the sample distribution of

$$\sum_{j=1}^{N} (X_j - \overline{X})^2 / \tau^2$$

has a χ^2 distribution with $N - 1$ degrees of freedom. According to Lehmann (1959), we can construct a $(1 - \alpha)100\%$ one-sided confidence interval for τ^2 as follows:

$$\tau^2 \geq \frac{\sum\limits_{j=1}^{N} (X_i - \overline{X})^2}{\chi^2(\alpha, N-1)}$$

$$= \xi.$$

We can reject the null hypothesis (Equation 10.3) and conclude that the items are not reliable in the estimation of θ if $\xi > \Delta$.

10.4.4 Ruggedness

In addition to validity and reliability, an acceptable TCM diagnostic instrument should produce similar results on different raters. In other words, it is desirable to quantify the variation owing to rater and the proportion of rater-to-rater variation to the total variation. We will use the one-way nested random model to evaluate the instrument ruggedness (Chow and Liu, 1995). The one-way nested random model can be expressed as

$$X_{ij} = \mu + A_i + e_{j(i)}, \quad i = 1 \text{ (Group 2), } 2 \text{ (Group 3), } j = 1, \dots, N,$$

where X_{ij} is the calibrated scale of the jth patient obtained from the ith rater, μ is the overall mean, A_i is the random effect owing to the ith rater, and $e_{j(i)}$ is the random error of jth patient's scale nested within the ith rater. For the one-way nested random model, we need the following assumptions: A_i are i.i.d. normal with mean 0 and variance σ_A^2; $e_{j(i)}$ are i.i.d. normal with mean 0 and variance σ^2; A_i and $e_{j(i)}$ are mutually independent for all i and j (Searle et al., 1992).

Let

$$\overline{X}_i = \frac{1}{J} \sum_{j=1}^{N} X_{ij} \quad \text{and} \quad \overline{X}_{..} = \frac{1}{2N} \sum_{i=1}^{2} \sum_{j=1}^{N} X_{ij} = \frac{1}{2} \sum_{i=1}^{2} \overline{X}_i$$

Let SSA and SSE denote the sum of squares of factor A and the sum of squares of errors, respectively. In other words,

$$\text{SSA} = N \sum_{i=1}^{2} \left(\overline{X}_{i\cdot} - \overline{X}_{\cdot\cdot} \right)^2$$

and

$$\text{SSE} = \sum_{i=1}^{2} \sum_{j=1}^{N} \left(X_{ij} - \overline{X}_{i\cdot} \right)^2.$$

Also, let MSA and MSE denote the mean squares for factor A and the mean square error, respectively. Then, MSA = SSA and MSE = $\text{SSE}/[2(N-1)]$. As a result, the analysis of variance estimators of σ_A^2 and σ^2 can be obtained as follows:

$$\hat{\sigma}^2 = \text{MSE}$$

and

$$\hat{\sigma}_A^2 = \frac{\text{MSA} - \text{MSE}}{N}.$$

Note that $\hat{\sigma}_A^2$ is obtained from the difference between MSA and MSE, and thus, it is possible to obtain a negative estimate for σ_A^2.

Three criteria can be used to evaluate instrument ruggedness. The first criterion is to compute the probability for obtaining a negative estimate of σ_A^2 given by

$$P\left(\hat{\sigma}_A^2 < 0\right) = P\left(F\left[1, 2(N-1)\right] < (F)^{-1}\right),$$

where $F[1, 2(N-1)]$ is a central F distribution with 1 and $2(N-1)$ degrees of freedom and

$$F = \frac{\sigma^2 + N\sigma_A^2}{\sigma^2}.$$

If $P\left(\hat{\sigma}_A^2 < 0\right)$ is large, it may suggest that $\sigma_A^2 = 0$. The second criterion is to test whether the variation owing to factor A is significantly > 0:

$$H_0: \sigma_A^2 = 0 \quad \text{versus} \quad H_1: \sigma_A^2 > 0. \tag{10.4}$$

The null hypothesis (Equation 10.4) is rejected at the α level of significance if

$$F_A > F_C = F(\alpha, 1, 2(N-1))$$

where $F_A = \text{MSA}/\text{MSE}$. The third criterion is to evaluate the proportion of the variation owing to factor A, which is defined as follows:

$$\rho_A = \frac{\sigma_A^2}{\sigma^2 + \sigma_A^2}.$$

By Searle et al. (1992), the estimator and the $(1-\alpha)100\%$ confidence interval for ρ_A are given by

$$\hat{\rho}_A = \frac{\text{MSA} - \text{MSE}}{\text{MSA} + (N-1)\text{MSE}},$$

$$L_\rho = \frac{F_A/F_U - 1}{N + (F_A/F_U - 1)},$$

$$U_\rho = \frac{F_A/F_L - 1}{N + (F_A/F_L - 1)},$$

where
$$F_L = F(1 - 0.5\alpha, 1, 2(N-1))$$
$$F_U = F(0.5\alpha, 1, 2(N-1))$$

It may be also desired to test whether or not the rater-to-rater variability is within an acceptable limit ω. With respect to this case, Hsiao et al. (2007) considered testing the following hypothesis:

$$H_0: \sigma_A^2 \geq \omega \quad \text{versus} \quad H_1: \sigma_A^2 < \omega. \tag{10.5}$$

Since there exists no exact $(1-\alpha)100\%$ confidence interval for σ_A^2, we can derive the Williams–Tukey interval with a confidence level between $(1-2\alpha)100\%$ and $(1-\alpha)100\%$, which is given by (L_A, U_A), where

$$L_A = \frac{\text{SSA}(1 - F_U/F_A)}{N\chi_{UA}^2},$$

$$U_A = \frac{\text{SSA}(1 - F_L/F_A)}{N\chi_{LA}^2},$$

where $F_L = F(1 - 0.5\alpha, 1, 2(N-1))$ and $F_U = F(0.5\alpha, 1, 2(N-1))$ represent the $(1 - 0.5\alpha)$th and (0.5α)th upper quantiles of a central F distribution with 1 and $2(N-1)$ degrees of freedom; $\chi_{LA}^2 = \chi^2(1 - 0.5\alpha, 1)$ and $\chi_{UA}^2 = \chi^2(0.5\alpha, 1)$ are the $(1 - 0.5\alpha)$th and (0.5α)th upper quantiles of a central χ^2 distribution with 1 degree of freedom; and $F_A = \text{MSA}/\text{MSE}$. The null hypothesis (Equation 10.5) is rejected at α level of significance if $U_A < \omega$.

10.4.5 Example

A modified data set taken from Chang Gung Memorial Hospital in Taiwan is used to illustrate the calibration and validation. The example is a randomized trial to study the effect of acupuncture for treating stroke patients. In this study, 30 stroke patients received aspirin and were evaluated by a Chinese doctor and a Western clinician (Group 1), 30 stroke patients received acupuncture and were evaluated by Chinese doctor A (Group 2), and 30 stroke patients received acupuncture and were evaluated by Chinese doctor B (Group 3). The measurement that the Western clinician used was the NIH Stroke Scale (NIHSS) developed by the U.S. National Institute of Neurological Disorder and Stroke (NINDS) from the original scale devised at the

TABLE 10.1: Wind and the fire-heat syndromes.

Wind Syndrome		Fire-Heat Syndrome	
Category	**Score**	**Category**	**Score**
Onset conditions	0–8	Tongue conditions	0–6
Limbs conditions	0–7	Tongue fur	0–5
Tongue body	0–7	Stool	0–4
Eyeballs conditions	0–3	Spirit	0–4
String-like pulse	0–3	Facial and breath conditions	0–3
Head conditions	0–2	Fever	0–3
		Pulse	0–2
		Mouth	0–2
		Urine	0–2

University of Cincinnati to measure the neurological impact of stroke, whereas the TCM diagnostic instruments considered in this study were wind and fire-heat syndromes. Table 10.1 summarizes the rating scales of the wind and fire-heat syndromes. The wind syndrome is a rating scale in 6 categories: onset conditions (score 0–8), limbs conditions (score 0–7), tongue body (score 0–7), eyeballs conditions (score 0–3), string-like pulse (score 0–3), and head conditions (score 0–2). Patients with a total score of > 7 were considered having wind syndrome. On the other hand, the fire-heat syndrome consists of 9 categories: tongue conditions (score 0–6), tongue fur (score 0–5), stool (score 0–4), spirit (score 0–4), facial and breath conditions (score 0–3), fever (score 0–3), pulse (score 0–2), mouth (score 0–2), and urine (score 0–1). Again, patients with a total score of >7 were considered to show fire-heat syndrome. The larger the scale is, the severer the syndrome is.

In this example, we summarize the TCM instruments based on the wind and fire-heat syndromes. That is, $K = 2$. From Group 1, the estimated standard curve based on the model 1 is given as

$$y = 7.358 + 1.861x,$$

where y represents the sum of the scores of wind and fire-heat syndromes and x represents the NIH stroke score. To provide better understanding, the estimated regression line as well as the original data is presented in Figure 10.2.

We use Group 2 to validate the CDP based on the previously established standard curve for calibration. In other words, we will claim that the instruments of wind and fire-heat syndromes are validated if

$$|\mu_i - \overline{\mu}| < \delta, \quad \forall i = 1, 2,$$

for some small prespecified δ. It can be seen from Group 2 that

$$\hat{\mu}_1 = 8.633 \quad \text{and} \quad \hat{\mu}_2 = 4.300.$$

The 95% simultaneous confidence intervals for $\mu_i - \overline{\mu}$ based on the Bonferroni adjustment are given by (1.249, 3.084) and (−3.084, −1.249), respectively. In this case, we cannot reject the null hypothesis (Equation 10.2) if $\delta = 0.5$.

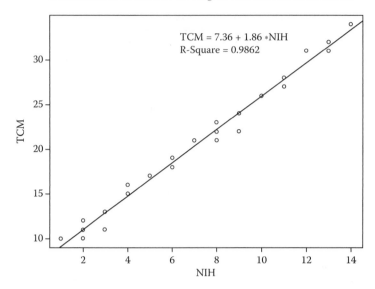

FIGURE 10.2: Scatter plot of data set in Group 1 and the estimated standard curve.

Group 2 is also used to evaluate the reliability of the items for the TCM instrument, i.e., the wind and fire-heat syndromes for the TCM instrument are considered reliable if the variance of X derived from the previously established standard curve is small. From Group 2, a 95% one-sided confidence interval for τ^2 can be constructed as follows:

$$\tau^2 \geq \frac{\sum\limits_{j=1}^{30} (X_j - \overline{X})^2}{\chi^2(0.05, 29)}$$
$$= \frac{27.13}{42.56}$$
$$= 0.64.$$

That is, $\xi = 0.64$. Therefore, we cannot reject the null hypothesis (Equation 10.3) if $\Delta = 1.0$ and conclude that the items are reliable. Selection of Δ should reflect the considerable information that existed in the previous studies.

Groups 2 and 3 are used to quantify the variation owing to raters. The ANOVA table is given in Table 10.2. From Table 10.2, it can be seen that

$$\text{SSA} = 190.778 \quad \text{and} \quad \text{SSE} = 77.244.$$

Hence, estimates for σ_A^2 and σ^2 are given by

$$\hat{\sigma}^2 = \text{MSE} = 1.332,$$
$$\hat{\sigma}_A^2 = \frac{\text{MSA} - \text{MSE}}{30} = \frac{190.778 - 1.332}{30} = 6.315.$$

TABLE 10.2: ANOVA table for the stroke data.

Source of Variation	Degrees of Freedom	Sum of Squares	Mean Square	F Value	p Value
Rater	1	190.778	190.778	143.25	<.0001
Error	58	77.244	1.332		
Total	59	268.022			

Since, $F_A = 0.274$ with a p value of < 0.0001, we may reject the null hypothesis (Equation 10.4) at the 5% level of significance. In addition, it can be verified that the probability for obtaining a negative estimate of σ_A^2 is given by

$$P\left(\hat{\sigma}_A^2 < 0\right) = P\left(F(1,58) < \frac{1}{143.25}\right) = 0.07.$$

The small probability for obtaining a negative rater-to-rater variation may suggest that there is greater rater-to-rater variation. That is, σ_A^2 might not be 0 and rater-to-rater variation may exist.

10.5 Concluding Remarks

In a TCM clinical trial, the validation of a standard quantitative instrument is critical to offer an accurate and reliable assessment of the safety and effectiveness of the TCM under investigation. Before the validation of CDP for the evaluation of TCM with respect to a well-established clinical endpoint for evaluation of WM, a calibration between the scale (or score) obtained from the CDP and the well-established clinical endpoint is necessary. Based on the calibration model, a detected difference by the CDP can be translated to the well-established clinical endpoint. In addition, the CDP can also be validated against the well-established clinical endpoint. This will provide the clinicians a better understanding of whether the detected significant difference from the quantitative instrument is clinically meaningful. On the basis of a well-calibrated and validated quantitative instrument, the sample size required for achieving a desired power for detecting a clinically meaningful difference can therefore be accurately estimated.

In some cases, validated quantitative TCM instruments for the diseases under study may not be available. In this case, a small-scale validation pilot study may be conducted to validate the quantitative instrument to be used in the intended clinical trials for a valid assessment of the safety and efficacy of the TCM under investigation. If such a small-scale pilot study is not feasible, a concurrent validation using a similar study design as described previously may be useful. In many situations, a retrospective validation may also be considered.

The use of TCM in humans for treating various diseases has a history of more than 5000 years, although no scientific documentations regarding clinical evidence of safety and efficacy of these TCMs are available. Though the use of TCM in humans has a long history, there are no regulatory requirements regarding the assessment of safety and effectiveness of the TCM until recently. For example, both the regulatory authorities of China and Taiwan have published guidelines/guidances for clinical development of TCMs (see, e.g., MOPH, 2002; DOH, 2004a,b). In addition, the United States Food and Drug Administration (FDA) also published a guidance for the botanical drug products (FDA, 2004). These regulatory requirements for TCM research and development, especially for clinical development are very similar to those well-established guidelines/guidances for pharmaceutical research and development of WM. It is a concern that whether these regulatory requirements are feasible for research and development of TCM, based on the fact that there are so many fundamental differences in medical practice, drug administration, and diagnostic procedure. As a result, it is suggested that current regulatory requirements should be modified to reflect these fundamental differences.

References

Chow, S. C. and Liu, J. P. 1995. *Statistical Design and Analysis in Pharmaceutical Science*. Marcel Dekker Inc., New York.

Chow, S. C., Pong, A., and Chang, Y. W. 2006. On traditional Chinese medicine clinical trials. *Drug Information Journal*, 40, 395–406.

DOH 2004a. *Draft Guidance for IND of Traditional Chinese Medicine*. The Department of Health, Taipei, Taiwan.

DOH 2004b. *Draft Guidance for NDA of Traditional Chinese Medicine*. The Department of Health, Taipei, Taiwan.

FDA 2004. Guidance for Industry—Botanical Drug Products. The United States Food and Drug Administration, Rockville, Maryland.

Hsiao, C. F., Tsou, H. H., Pong A., Liu J. P., Lin, C. H., and Chow, S. C. 2007. Statistical validation of traditional Chinese diagnostic procedure (under revision).

Lehmann, E. L. 1959. *Testing Statistical Hypotheses*. Wiley, New York.

MOPH 2002. Guidance for Drug Registration. Ministry of Public Health, Beijing, China.

Searle, S. R., Casella, G., and McCulloch, C. E. 1992. *Variance Components*. Wiley, New York.

Wu, L. 2000. Principles of Traditional Chinese Medicine, *Conscious Choice*, Traditional Chinese Medicine, December Issue.

Wu, T., Zhao, N., Liu, G., and Ni, J. 2004. A huge challenge: Traditional Chinese medicine vs. Cochrane systematic review, *Cochrane Colloquia*, Ottawa, Canada.

Index